# MEMORY BANK
## FOR
# MEDICATIONS

By Christina L.S. Evans
RNC, MSN, CNA

# MEMORY BANK

# FOR

# MEDICATIONS

By Christina L.S. Evans
RNC, MSN, CNA

A NURSECO BOOK

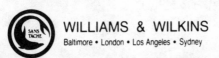

WILLIAMS & WILKINS
Baltimore • London • Los Angeles • Sydney

*Printed in the United States of America*

**Library of Congress Cataloging in Publication Data**

Evans, Christina L.S.
Memory bank for medications

    "A Nurseco book."
    Bibliography: p.
    1. Drugs—Outlines, syllabi, etc.  2. Nursing—Outlines, syllabi, etc.  I. Title [DNLM: 1. Drugs—nurses' instruction. QV 55 E925m]
RM301.E9    1985    615.1    84-18893
ISBN 0-683-09545-5

89  88  87  86  85

10  9  8  7  6  5  4  3  2  1

# Notice

Clinical health care is a dynamic field because of the continuous availability of new information. Eventually this new information may lead to necessary changes in treatment methodology and the use of drugs. The author and the publisher of *Memory Bank for Medications* have carefully reviewed doses of drugs and treatment modalities for correct content and compatibility with general standards of care acceptable at the time of publication. Before administering a drug, review instructions and information on the manufacturer's package insert to verify that recommended dosage is correct and unchanged, and that no changes have occurred related to uses or contraindications of the drug. (This review is always advisable, and especially when using a new or infrequently used drug.)

---

The author and publisher wish to thank
Robert F. Stankiewicz, RPh,
Coordinator, Department of Pharmacy Services,
Henry Ford Hospital,
for his assistance in the preparation
of this manuscript.

---

# Contents

# Preface

*Memory Bank for Medications* was written to assist nurses to increase their independent decision-making regarding the dependent action of administering medications.

The idea for the book was conceived from the experience of working with students and RNs. These nurses were facing an overwhelming task—that of sorting through an immense amount of pharmaceutical data to make it into a comprehensible entity. The format of *Memory Bank for Medications* does just that: it presents the most important information on each drug and presents it in an easy-to-read way.

*Memory Bank for Medications* is not designed to be a prescriptive text but an informational resource. It does not include all information regarding a medication; it is intended for use as a convenient resource text. For additional information, or clarification, refer to the Physicians' Desk Reference, the manufacturer's literature, or other pharmacology texts.

The uses, doses, and other drug information presented in this publication are based on research and consultation with pharmaceutical and nursing authorities. To the best of our knowledge, this information reflects currently accepted clinical practice; nevertheless, it cannot be considered absolute. For individual application, recommendations must be considered in light of the patient's clinical condition. Before administration of new or infrequently used drugs, review of the patient's medication profile and consultation with physician and/or the pharmacist is advised. The author disclaims responsibility for any adverse effects resulting directly or indirectly from the suggested procedures or from the reader's misunderstanding of the text.

Christina L. S. Evans

# Format Explanation

**Brand Name**
Selected brand names; most common one is listed first; the rest in alphabetical order.

**Actions**
Drug classification(s) and methods by which the medication causes its effects; not always known. Includes time of onset as known.

**Uses**
Disease processes for which the medication is prescribed.

**Contraindications**
Medications, conditions, diseases with which the medication should not be used or should be used cautiously. When a pediatric dose is not listed, *extreme caution* should be exercised if the medication is ordered for a child.

**Interactions**
The most common medications that interact with the drug.

**Dose**
General dosage ranges for adult and pediatric patients; many contain recommended doses for initial, maximum, and maintenance doses. Doses listed are generally for the oral route; refer to other pharmacologic resources for parenteral doses not otherwise specified. Adult doses must be individualized for older children if the medication is not contraindicated.

**Forms**
Available forms of the drug

## Adverse Effects
Alphabetized list of common side effects that may occur

## Special Nursing Considerations and Patient Education
- General considerations for administration of the medication.
- What to monitor during the course of treatment with the medication.
- Facts relevant to patient education. Rationales are generally not included. Refer to other pharmacology texts for additional information.

# Part I
# Medications

# Acetaminophen

**Brand Name**
Tylenol, Datril, Tempra

**Actions**
Analgesic, antipyretic; elevates pain threshold; affects heat-regulating aspect of hypothalamus

**Uses**
Fever, pain

**Contraindications**
Anemia, glucose-6-phosphate dehydrogenase deficiencies; cardiac or pulmonary disease

**Interactions**
Coumarin anticoagulants

**Dose**
*Adult*  PO: 325–650 mg q4–6h to a *maximum* of 4 gm/day
*Peds*  PO: 3–6 yr: 120 mg tid–qid
7–12 yr: 162–325 mg tid–qid

**Forms**
Capsules, chewable tablets, elixirs, suppositories, tablets

**Adverse Effects**
Abdominal pain, nausea, vomiting; toxic doses can cause hepatic and renal tubular necrosis

**Special Nursing Considerations
and Patient Education**
- Protect medication from direct light.
- Use as aspirin substitute to relieve pain and fever especially for patients with a viral infection.
- Be aware that
  - medication causes fewer GI adverse effects than aspirin.
  - this drug does not have anti-inflammatory effects and cannot replace aspirin in these cases.
  - it is safe at usual doses for use during lactation.

# Acetazolamide

**Brand Name**
Diamox

**Actions**
Diuretic, carbonic anhydrase inhibitor (lessens concentration of hydrogen ions in tubules). Onset evident in 2 hours.

**Uses**
Chronic simple glaucoma, congestive heart failure, convulsive disorders, edema

**Contraindications**
Addison's disease, chronic noncongestive angle-closure glaucoma, hepatic disease, hyperchloremic acidosis, low serum levels of potassium and sodium, renal disease, supra-renal gland disease.
*Use with caution:* past allergic reactions to sulfa drugs, diabetes, gout, lupus erythematosus

**Interactions**
Amphetamines, lithium, methenamine salts, oral hypoglycemics, quinidine, theophylline, tricyclic antidepressants

**Dose**
*Adult*  PO: 250 mg–1 gm/day
*Peds*   PO: 5 mg/kg/day

**Forms**
Injection, sequels, tablets

**Adverse Effects**
Anorexia, confusion, drowsiness, hematuria, hypokalemia, paresthesia, polyuria, unusual bleeding, urticaria

**Special Nursing Considerations
and Patient Education**
- Monitor urinary output, weight.
- Include potassium-rich foods in patient's diet (see Appendix F).
- Discontinue if electrolyte imbalance or allergic signs are evident.
- Be aware that
  - IV route is less painful than IM injection.
  - drug's effectiveness lessens after 2 days.
  - tolerance can develop.
- Teach patient
  - that medication may cause drowsiness and confusion.
  - to notify physician if tingling feeling in hands and feet, loss of appetite, fever, rash, unusual bleeding, or bruising occurs.

# Acetohexamide

**Brand Name**
Dymelor

**Actions**
Stimulates secretion of insulin

**Uses**
Oral antidiabetic

**Contraindications**
*Meds* Alcohol
*Other* Diabetic conditions complicated by acidosis,
coma, infection, trauma, controlled by diet, or
insulin-dependent diabetes; patients with
hepatic, renal, or thyroid dysfunction. *Use with
caution:* peptic ulcer, porphyria

**Interactions**
Anti-inflammatory agents, barbiturates,
chloramphenicol clofibrate, cortisone, coumarin
anticoagulants, estrogens, hypnotics, isoniazid,
MAO inhibitors, nicotinic acid, oral contraceptives,
oxyphenbutazone, phenylbutazone, propranolol,
salicylates, sedatives, sulfa medications, thiazide
diuretics, thyroid preparations

**Dose**
*Adult* 250 mg–1.5 gm/day

**Forms**
Tablets

**Adverse Effects**
Diarrhea, headache, hypoglycemia, jaundice,
nausea

## Special Nursing Considerations and Patient Education
- Teach patient
  - to follow prescribed diet.
  - to be alert for symptoms of hypo- and hyperglycemia (see Appendix B).
  - that medication may cause photosensitivity.
  - to be cautious with strenuous exercise since this may require dose adjustments in the medication.
  - to notify physician of illness.
  - to take medication at meal time or with food or milk to minimize gastric irritation.

# Acetylcysteine

**Brand Name**
Mucomyst

**Actions**
Expectorant, mucolytic; disrupts disulfide linkages in mucus

**Uses**
Adjuvant therapy for patients with abnormal, viscid, or inspissated mucus secretions in such conditions as anesthesia, bronchial studies, bronchopulmonary disorders, cystic fibrosis with pulmonary complications

**Contraindications**
None

**Interactions**
Asthma

**Dose**
*Adult* 3-5 cc of 20% solution or 6-10 cc of 10% solution tid-qid
*Peds* Same as adult

**Forms**
Solution

**Adverse Effects**
Bronchospasm, chills and fever, hemoptysis, nausea, rhinorrhea, stomatitis

## Special Nursing Considerations
## and Patient Education

- Have bronchodilators available in case of bronchospasm.
- Wash patient's face after use with a mask.
- Be aware that
  - solution hardens and becomes discolored when in contact with specific metals.
  - if solution turns purple, it is not harmful.
- Teach patient
  - that nauseous odors will decrease in intensity.

# Alcohol/Diphenhydramine HCl

**Brand Name**
  Benylin

**Actions**
  Antihistamine, antitussive

**Uses**
  Cough relief

**Contraindications**
*Meds*  MAO inhibitors
*Other*  Asthma, bladder-neck or pyloroduodenal
  obstructions, narrow-angle glaucoma,
  neonates, premature infants, prostatic
  hypertrophy, stenosing peptic ulcer.
  *Use with caution:* asthma

**Interactions**
  Alcohol, CNS depressants

**Dose**
*Adult*  25–50 mg tid–qid; *maximum* dose: 400 mg/day
*Peds*  5 mg/kg/day, in 4 divided doses; *maximum*
  dose: 300 mg/day

**Forms**
  Syrup

**Adverse Effects**
  Blurred vision, confusion, constipation, diarrhea,
  drowsiness, dry mouth, hypotension, nausea,
  nervousness, restlessness, vomiting

**Special Nursing Considerations
and Patient Education**
- Protect medication from direct light.
- Offer hard candy (regular or sugar-free) to relieve dry mouth.
- Teach patient
  - that medication may cause photosensitivity.
  - to keep syrup out of reach of children.
  - to change position slowly to decrease possibility of hypotension.
  - to be cautious when driving or involved in potentially hazardous tasks.
  - to take with meals or milk to decrease GI upset.

# Allopurinol

**Brand Name**
Zyloprim, Lopurim

**Actions**
Controls hyperuricemia. Onset evident in 24–48 hours.

**Uses**
Gout, recurrent uric-acid stone formation, uric-acid nephropathy

**Contraindications**
*Meds* Iron preparations
*Other* Children (unless as an adjunct with chemo-therapy), idiopathic hemochromatosis. *Use with caution:* History of hepatic or renal disease

**Interactions**
Anticoagulants, azathioprine, mercaptopurine, theophylline, uricosuric agents

**Dose**
*Adult* 200–600 mg/day in divided doses
*Peds* Under 6 yr: 50 mg tid
6–10 yr: 100 mg tid

**Forms**
Tablets

**Adverse Effects**
Alopecia, diarrhea, drowsiness, nausea, pruritus, rash, vomiting

## Special Nursing Considerations and Patient Education

- Give amounts of 300 mg in 1 dose.
- Reduce dose in renal failure.
- Transfer from other medications gradually.
- Monitor blood counts, I&O.
- Teach patient to
  - keep well hydrated (2,000 cc/day).
  - take each dose with full glass of water; if GI upset occurs, take with food.
  - be cautious when driving or involved in potentially hazardous tasks.
  - discontinue if rash occurs.

# Alprazolam

**Brand Name**
Xanax

**Actions**
CNS depressant

**Uses**
Anxiety; *not* of value in treatment of psychoses

**Contraindications**
*Meds* Alcohol, hypersensitivity to benzodiazepines
*Other* Acute narrow-angle glaucoma, children under
18. *Use with caution:* Hepatic or renal
impairment

**Interactions**
Anticonvulsants, antihistamines, barbiturates,
cimetidine, CNS depressants, hypnotics, narcotics,
oral anticoagulants, sedatives, tranquilizers

**Dose**
*Adult* 0.25–5 mg tid; *maximum* dose: 4 mg/day in
divided doses

**Forms**
Tablets

**Adverse Effects**
Confusion, constipation, depression, diarrhea,
drowsiness, dry mouth, headache, light-
headedness, nausea, vomiting

**Special Nursing Considerations
and Patient Education**
- Use caution when administering to patients with
  suicidal potential; ensure patient swallows dose.
- Monitor patient's physical and mental status
  periodically.
- Be aware that
  - Habituation and dependence are possible; when
    discontinued, decrease dosage gradually.
- Teach patient
  - that effects may continue after treatment ends.
  - to be cautious when driving or involved in
    potentially hazardous tasks.
  - to avoid alcohol and other CNS depressants.

# Aminocaproic Acid

**Brand Name**
Amicar

**Actions**
Fibrinolytic inhibitor, systemic hemostatic; reduces plasminogen activator substances and demonstrates antiplasmin activity

**Uses**
Treatment of excessive bleeding resulting from systemic hyperfibrinolysis and urinary fibrinolysis; used investigationally to prevent recurrence of subarachnoid hemorrhage

**Contraindications**
Active intravascular clotting process (not used unless there is definite diagnosis of hyperfibrinolysis). *Use with caution:* Cardiac, hepatic, or renal dysfunction; uremia

**Interactions**
Estrogens, oral contraceptives, probenecid

**Dose**
*Adult*  PO: Initial dose: 4–5 gm; then, 1–1.25 gm/hr for 8 hr or until bleeding is controlled
*Peds*  PO: 100 mg/kg q6h for 6 days

**Forms**
Injection, syrup, tablets

**Adverse Effects**
Bradycardia, dysrhythmias, hypotension (IV use); conjunctival suffusion; cramps; diarrhea; dizziness; headache; malaise; nasal stuffiness; nausea; rash; tinnitus

**Special Nursing Considerations
and Patient Education**
- Give IV slowly.
- Monitor plasma levels, potassium, vital signs.
- Be aware that
  - optimal plasma level is 0.130 mg/cc.
  - medication may elevate serum potassium levels.

# Aminophylline

**Brand Name**
Somophyllin

**Actions**
Bronchodilator, decongestant; inhibits phosphodiesterase which leads to increased epinephrine

**Uses**
Bronchial asthma, cardiac paroxysmal dyspnea, Cheyne-Stokes respirations, congestive heart failure, emphysema, pulmonary edema, status asthmaticus

**Contraindications**
Hypersensitivity to any xanthine; rectal suppositories contraindicated in presence of irritation or infection of rectum or lower colon. *Use with caution:* Cardiac, hepatic, or renal dysfunction; coronary artery disease; hypertension; hyperthyroid; MI; peptic ulcer; porphyria; prostatic hypertrophy

**Interactions**
Beta-blocking agents, tetracycline, reserpine, chlordiazepoxide; *effects decreased* by cigarette smoke, phenobarbital; *effects increased* by allopurinol, cimetidine, clindamycin, influenza vaccine, lincomycin, thiabendazole; *increases* effects of adrenergics, digitalis, furosemide, oral anticoagulants; *decreases* effects of lithium, phenytoin. Medication is incompatible with many IV drugs.

## Dose

*Adult* PO: 100–315 mg q6–8h
*Peds* PO: 3.5–5 mg/kg q6–8h

## Forms

Elixir, extended-action tablets, injection, oral liquid, rectal solution, suppository, tablets

## Adverse Effects

Diarrhea, dizziness, extrasystoles, flushing, generalized convulsions, headache, hypotension, irritability, nausea, palpitations, restlessness, tachypnea, vomiting

## Special Nursing Considerations and Patient Education

- Warm IV solutions to body temperature, dilute, give slowly.
- Give oral forms with glass of water on an empty stomach 1 hour before or 2 hours after meals.
- Administer on a regular basis over 24 hours.
- Monitor vital signs.
- Maintain plasma levels at 10–20 $\mu$g/cc.
- Be aware that
  - IM injection is very painful.
- Teach patient
  - to be cautious when driving or involved in potentially hazardous tasks.
  - to notify physician of cramps, dizziness, headache, insomnia, palpitations, stomach upset.
  - that smoking may decrease effectiveness of medication.

# Aminosalicylic Acid
# (Para-Aminosalicylic Acid)

**Brand Name**
PAS

**Actions**
Antitubercular, bacteriostatic; delays tubercle resistance to isoniazid and streptomycin

**Uses**
Adjunct in treatment of extrapulmonary and pulmonary tuberculosis

**Contraindications**
*Meds* Salicylates
*Other* Renal dysfunction. *Use with caution:* Peptic ulcer

**Interactions**
Ammonium chloride, digitalis, isoniazid, oral anticoagulants, phenytoin, probenecid, pyrazinamide, rifampin

**Dose**
*Adult* 8–15 gm/day in 2–4 equal doses
*Peds* 200–300 mg/kg/day in equal doses

**Forms**
Buffered tablets, enteric-coated tablets, resins, tablets, solutions

**Adverse Effects**
Abdominal pain, acidosis, agranulocytosis, anorexia, diarrhea, eosinophilia, hypokalemia, leukopenia, nausea, rash, vomiting

**Special Nursing Considerations
and Patient Education**
- Teach patient
  - to store medication away from moisture.
  - to use oral solutions within 24 hours.
  - to discard medication if it has brown or purple coloring.
  - to use Tes-Tape to test urine of diabetic patient.
  - that medication may cause a peculiar taste in mouth.
  - to keep well hydrated.
  - to avoid medications or foods that acidify urine (e.g., cranberry juice).
  - to take oral forms after meals to help decrease GI distress.
  - that medication may cause abnormal discoloration of urine.
  - to discontinue medication for unusual bleeding, fever, rash, sore throat, peculiar taste in mouth.

# Amitriptyline HCl

**Brand Name**
Elavil, Endep, Etrafon

**Actions**
Tricyclic antidepressant; affects central nervous system. Onset evident in 1-2 weeks.

**Uses**
Depression, enuresis (children)

**Contraindications**
*Meds* Alcohol, ethchlorvynol, MAO inhibitors, procainamide, quinidine, reserpine, thyroid preparations

*Other* Closed-angle glaucoma, MI, prostatic hypertrophy, pyloric stenosis, renal dysfunction, urinary retention. *Use with caution:* Asthma, diabetes, epilepsy, GI and hepatic disorders

**Interactions**
Adrenergics, amphetamines, anticholinergics, anticonvulsants, antihistamines, beta-blockers, clonidine, CNS depressants, guanethidine, levodopa, narcotics, oral coumarins, sedatives, tranquilizers dysfunction, hyperthyroidism

**Dose**
*Adult* PO: 10-25 mg bid-qid (hospitalized patients may need as much as 300 mg/day)
*Peds* PO: Adolescent: 10 mg tid with 20 mg at hs

**Forms**
Injection, tablets

## Adverse Effects

Anorexia, blurred vision, dizziness, drowsiness, dry mouth, headache, nausea, peculiar taste, orthostatic hypotension, vomiting

## Special Nursing Considerations and Patient Education

- Decrease dosage slowly.
- Teach patient
  - that medicine may cause urine to be colored blue-green, and may cause photosensitivity.
  - to be cautious when driving or involved in potentially hazardous tasks.
  - not to take other medications without consulting with physician.
  - to avoid alcohol.

# Amobarbital, Amobarbital Sodium

**Brand Name**
Amytal, Tuinal

**Actions**
Hypnotic, sedative. Onset evident in 30–60 minutes.

**Uses**
Acute convulsive disorders, insomnia

**Contraindications**
*Meds* Alcohol, CNS depressants
*Other* History of porphyria; renal dysfunction; uncontrolled pain. *Use with caution:* Asthma, borderline hypoadrenalism, cardiac dysfunction, hepatic or pulmonary dysfunction, hypertension (IM/IV use), hypotension, hypothyroidism, respiratory distress

**Interactions**
Antidepressants, beta-blockers, cortisone, digitalis, griseofulvin, MAO inhibitors, narcotics, oral anti-coagulants, oral contraceptives, phenylbutazone, phenytoin, quinidine, tetracycline, valproic acid

**Dose**
*Adult* PO: Hypnotic: 100–200 mg; sedative: 30–50 mg bid-tid
*Peds* PO: 3–6 mg/kg/day in 3 equal doses

**Forms**
Capsules, elixir, sodium salt injection, tablets

**Adverse Effects**
Ataxia, dizziness, emotional disturbances, excitement, lethargy, nausea, pruritus, restlessness

**Special Nursing Considerations and Patient Education**

- Medication is addictive; when discontinued, decrease dosage gradually.
- Inject IM doses into deep muscle; give no more than 5 cc at one site.
- Monitor vital signs closely when giving IV; *maximum* IV rate is 1 cc/minute.
- When used as a hypnotic, administer 30–60 minutes before hs.
- Teach patient
  - that medication can lower body temperature; if elderly, to be cautious during cold weather.
  - that medication may cause photosensitivity.
  - to be cautious when driving or involved in potentially hazardous tasks.
  - to avoid alcohol.

# Amphetamine Sulfate

**Brand Name**
  Benzedrine

**Actions**
  Sympathomimetic amines with CNS stimulant
  activity

**Uses**
  Behavior problems in children, exogenous obesity,
  narcolepsy

**Contraindications**
  MAO inhibitors
  *Use with caution:* Agitated states, arteriosclerosis,
  cardiovascular dysfunction, drug abuse, glaucoma,
  hypertension, hyperthyroidism, psychoses

**Interactions**
  Anesthetics, antihypertensives, insulin, phenothiazines, tricyclic antidepressants, urinary alkalizers

**Dose**
*Adult*  5–60 mg/day in divided doses
*Peds*  3–5 yr: 2.5 mg/day
      6–12 yr: 5 mg/day
      over 12 yr: 10 mg/day

**Forms**
  Sustained-release capsules, tablets

**Adverse Effects**
  Anorexia, blurred vision, constipation, dizziness,
  dry mouth, headache, hypertension, insomnia,
  irritability, nervousness, psychotic episodes,
  restlessness, tachycardia

## Special Nursing Considerations and Patient Education

- Give sustained-release form in morning.
- When used for obesity, give 30 to 60 minutes before meals.
- Do not crush capsules.
- Offer hard candy (regular or sugar-free) to relieve dry mouth.
- Be aware that
  - medication may affect insulin requirements in patients with diabetes.
  - habituation and dependence are possible; when discontinued, decrease dose gradually.
- Teach patient to
  - obtain adequate rest despite feelings of high energy.
  - be cautious when driving or involved in potentially hazardous tasks.

# Ampicillin, Ampicillin Sodium

**Brand Name**
  Polycillin, Amcill, Omnipen, SK-Ampicillin

**Actions**
  Interferes with ability of susceptible bacteria to create cell walls as they multiply and grow

**Uses**
  Endocarditis; meningitis; respiratory tract, skin, soft tissue, and urinary tract infections

**Contraindications**
*Meds*  Hypersensitivity to penicillins or cephalosporins
*Other*  Infectious mononucleosis. *Use with caution:* Renal failure

**Interactions**
  Bacteriostatic antibiotics (erythromycin, tetracycline), oral contraceptives, probenecid

**Dose**
*Adult*  PO: 250–500 mg q6h
*Peds*  PO: 25–50 mg/kg/day in divided doses q6–8h

**Forms**
  Chewable tablets, pediatric drops, sodium salt injection, trihydrate capsules or suspension

**Adverse Effects**
  Dark discoloration of tongue, diarrhea, glossitis, nausea, nephritis, stomatitis, superinfections, urticaria

## Special Nursing Considerations and Patient Education
- Refrigerate liquid forms.
- Inject IV form slowly (2 cc/3–5 minutes).
- Monitor urinary output.
- Administer oral forms 1 hour before or 2 hours after meals.
- If an outpatient, have patient remain in office for 30 minutes after receiving medication for first time.
- Inspect skin frequently for signs of rash.
- Be aware that
  - a cross reaction is possible if patient is hypersensitive to cephalosporins.
- Teach patient
  - to take entire prescription.

# Amyl Nitrite

**Actions**
Antianginal, coronary vasodilator. Onset evident in 30 seconds.

**Uses**
Angina pectoris, antidote for cyanide poisoning

**Contraindications**
Cerebral hemorrhage, head trauma

**Interactions**
None

**Dose**
*Adult* 0.18–0.3 cc prn

**Forms**
Inhaler

**Adverse Effects**
Flushing, headache, hypotension, nausea, reflex tachycardia, syncope, vomiting

**Special Nursing Considerations
and Patient Education**
- Be aware that
  - medication has strong unpleasant odor.
- Teach patient
  - that medication is flammable.
  - correct usage of inhaler: sit down and take deep
    breaths.

# Aspirin

**Brand Name**
ASA, Ecotrin, Empirin

**Actions**
Analgesic (raises pain threshold), anti-inflammatory, antipyretic (affects heat-regulatory center of hypothalamus). Onset evident in 15–20 minutes.

**Uses**
Fever, relief of mild to moderate pain, rheumatic fever, rheumatoid arthritis

**Contraindications**
*Meds* Anticoagulants, ulcerogenics
*Other* Active ulcers, tendency to hemorrhage. *Use with caution:* Anemia, asthma, diabetes, hepatic or renal dysfunction, history of ulcers or gout, Hodgkin's disease, hypoprothrombinemia, viral infection

**Interactions**
Alcohol, antacids, furosemide, methotrexate, oral anticoagulants, phenylbutazone, probenecid, spironolactone, steroids, sulfinpyrazone, urinary acidifiers

**Dose**
*Adult* PO: 325–650 mg q3–4h
*Peds* PO: 65 mg/kg/day in divided doses q6h

**Forms**
Capsules, children's tablets, enteric-coated tablets, suppository, tablets

## Adverse Effects

Asthma, GI bleeding, indigestion, nausea, tarry stools, vomiting

## Special Nursing Considerations and Patient Education

- Do not administer if it has a vinegar odor.
- If stomach upset occurs, try a different brand.
- Be aware that
  - medication may cause false positive urine-glucose tests.
  - aspirin should not be given to patients with a viral infection (may lead to Reye's syndrome).
- Teach patient to
  - assess aspirin content of other current medications.
  - notify physician of ringing in ears or persistent GI pain.
  - keep out of reach of children.
  - take with full glass of water or milk.

# Aspirin/Butalbital/Caffeine

**Brand Name**
  Fiorinal

**Actions**
  Analgesic, antipyretic

**Uses**
  Tension headache

**Contraindications**
  Children under 12, porphyria. *Use with caution:*
  Coagulation disorders, peptic ulcer, viral
  infections.

**Interactions**
  Alcohol, hypnotics, sedatives

**Dose**
*Adult* 1–2 tablets q4h; *maximum* dose: 6 tablets/day

**Forms**
  Tablets

**Adverse Effects**
  Dizziness, drowsiness, GI distress,
  light-headedness

**Special Nursing Considerations
and Patient Education**
- Administer with meals to decrease irritation.
- When discontinued, decrease dosage gradually.
- Be aware that
  - dependence is possible.
- Teach patient
  - to be cautious when driving or involved in
    potentially hazardous tasks.

# Aspirin/Caffeine/ Orphenadrine Citrate

**Brand Name**
Norgesic, Norgesic Forte

**Actions**
Skeletal muscle relaxant

**Uses**
Acute painful musculoskeletal conditions, parkinsonism

**Contraindications**
Achalasia, cardiospasm, glaucoma, intestinal obstruction, myasthenia gravis, urinary retention; children under 12. *Use with caution:* Renal disorders, tachycardia, viral infections

**Interactions**
Alcohol, CNS depressants

**Dose**
*Adult* ½–2 tablets tid–qid

**Forms**
Tablets

**Adverse Effects**
Blurred vision, constipation, dizziness, drowsiness, dry mouth, headache, increased ocular tension, nausea, nephrotoxicity, palpitation, pruritus, pupil dilation, tachycardia, vomiting

## Special Nursing Considerations and Patient Education

- Offer hard candy (regular or sugar-free) to relieve dry mouth.
- Increase fluid and bulk intake to help relieve constipation.
- Teach patient
  - to be cautious when driving or involved in potentially hazardous tasks.

# Atropine Sulfate

## Actions

Anticholinergic, antispasmodic, mydriatic. Onset evident in 1-2 hours.

## Uses

Bradycardia, bronchial asthma, cardiospasm, colitis, dysmenorrhea, enuresis, GI spasm, paralysis agitans, parkinsonism, pylorospasm, rigid/spastic conditions caused by CNS injury, ureteral colic, urinary frequency

## Contraindications

Adhesions between iris and lens, hepatic or renal dysfunction, intestinal atony, myasthenia gravis, narrow-angle glaucoma, obstructive conditions of GI and urinary tract, reflex esophagitis, ulcerative colitis. *Use with caution:* Angina, chronic bronchitis, debilitated patients with chronic lung disease, hiatal hernia, prostatic hypertrophy, tachycardia

## Interactions

Antacids, anticholinergics, antihistamines, guanethidine, haloperidol, MAO inhibitors, methylphenidate, nitrates, primidone, procainamide, quinidine, reserpine

## Dose

*Adult*  PO: 0.4-0.6 mg q4-6h
Peds  PO: 0.01 mg/kg q4-6h

## Forms

Injection, ophthalmic ointment or solution, tablets

## Adverse Effects

Blurred vision, constipation, cycloplegia, dry mouth, flushing, increased intraocular pressure, mydriasis, nausea, suppression of body secretions, vomiting

## Special Nursing Considerations and Patient Education

- Store in light-resistant containers.
- Monitor vital signs.
- Offer hard candy (regular or sugar-free) to relieve dry mouth.
- Provide increased fluids and bulk in diet to ease constipation.
- Administer tablets 30 minutes before meals.
- Discontinue for eye pain, flushing, rash.
- Teach patient
  - to avoid strenuous work in hot weather to prevent heat stroke.
  - to be cautious when driving or involved in potentially hazardous tasks.

# Azathioprine

**Brand Name**
Imuran

**Actions**
Immunosuppressant; interferes with utilization of purine by cell

**Uses**
Autoimmune hemolytic anemia, idiopathic thrombocytopenic purpura, rheumatoid arthritis, systemic lupus erythematosus

**Contraindications**
*Meds* Live vaccinations
*Other* Biliary stasis, pre-existing or drug-induced bone-marrow suppression, toxic hepatitis.
*Use with caution:* Gout, hepatic or renal dysfunction, infection, pancreatitis, radiation

**Interactions**
Allopurinol, corticosteroids, myelosuppressive agents

**Dose**
*Adult* PO: Individualized: 3–5 mg/kg/day

**Forms**
Powder (for injection), tablets

**Adverse Effects**
Alopecia, arthralgia, fever, hepatitis, infection, leukopenia, nausea, pulmonary edema, rashes, thrombocytopenia, vomiting

## Special Nursing Considerations
## and Patient Education
- Store medication in light-resistant containers.
- Observe for rejection of transplant, if applicable.
- Monitor CBC (particularly platelets), I&O, renal clearance, weight.
- Offer bland foods to reduce nausea.
- Be aware that
  - medication is highly toxic.
- Teach patient to
  - decrease fruit juice intake if diarrhea occurs.
  - to use birth control during and for 4 months after treatment.
  - take precautions to avoid infections.
  - notify physician for unusual bleeding, fever, infection, sore throat.

# Bacitracin

**Actions**
Antibacterial, antibiotic, anti-infective; inhibits cell wall synthesis in susceptible microorganisms

**Uses**
Limited to treatment of infants with pneumonia and empyema caused by staphylococci

**Contraindications**
Colistimethate sodium, kanamycin, neomycin, polymyxin-B, streptomycin, topical or systemic nephrotoxics, viomycin

**Interactions**
None

**Dose**
*Peds* Under 2.5 kg: 900 U/kg/day in 2–3 divided doses; over 2.5 kg: 1,000 U/kg/day in 2–3 divided doses

**Forms**
Injection

**Adverse Effects**
None

## Special Nursing Considerations and Patient Education

- Dissolve in sodium chloride containing 2% procaine hydrochloride.
- Rotate IM sites and administer in upper, outer quadrant of buttocks.
- Monitor I&O, renal function, urine pH.
- Be aware that
  - injection is painful.

# Baclofen

**Brand Name**
Lioresal

**Actions**
Antispasmodic, muscle relaxant; inhibits neural transmissions in spinal cord

**Uses**
Multiple sclerosis spasticity, spinal cord injuries and diseases

**Contraindications**
*Meds* Alcohol, CNS depressants
*Other* Children under 12, CVA; *Use with caution:* diabetes, epilepsy, renal dysfunction

**Interactions**
Hypoglycemics, insulin, MAO inhibitors, tricyclic antidepressants

**Dose**
*Adult* Start at 5 mg tid; increase by 5 mg q3days until optimum effect is achieved; *maximum:* 80 mg/day

**Forms**
Tablets

**Adverse Effects**
Abdominal pain, anorexia, chest pain, confusion, constipation, dizziness, drowsiness, fatigue, hallucinations, headache, hematuria, hypotension, insomnia, nasal congestion, nausea, pruritus, urinary frequency, weakness

**Special Nursing Considerations
and Patient Education**
• When discontinued, decrease dosage gradually.
• Be aware that
  – if patient is diabetic, medication may cause an
    increase of glucose in the urine.
  – spasticity is necessary to maintain balance,
    locomotion, and posture in certain diseases.
• Teach patient to
  – be cautious when driving or involved in
    potentially hazardous tasks.
  – avoid alcohol and other CNS depressants.

# Benzquinamide HCl

**Brand Name**
Emete-Con

**Actions**
Antiemetic; depresses chemoreceptor trigger zone in medulla

**Uses**
Nausea and vomiting associated with anesthesia and surgery

**Contraindications**
Cardiovascular disease (IV dose), children under 12

**Interactions**
Epinephrine

**Dose**
*Adult* IM: 0.5–1 mg/kg q3–4h

**Forms**
Powder (for injection)

**Adverse Effects**
Anorexia, atrial fibrillation, blurred vision, diaphoresis, drowsiness, excitement, headache, hiccoughs, hypertension, hypotension, insomnia, nervousness, shivering

## Special Nursing Considerations and Patient Education
- Store in light-resistant containers.
- Monitor blood pressure after IV dose.
- Administer IM dose into large muscle.
- Be aware that
  - drug may mask toxicity of other medications being used.

# Benztropine Mesylate

**Brand Name**
Cogentin

**Actions**
Anticholinergic; hinders synaptic transmissions in cholinergic neurons in CNS. Onset evident in 2–3 days.

**Uses**
Adjunct therapy of all forms of parkinsonism; used in control of extrapyramidal disorders (except tardive dyskinesia) resulting from neuroleptic drugs (e.g., phenothiazines)

**Contraindications**
*Meds*  Alcohol, nonprescription cough/hay fever preparations
*Other*  Children under 3, closed-angle glaucoma. *Use with caution:* Atropine sensitivity, cardiovascular disease, children over 3, glaucoma, hepatic or renal dysfunction, hypertension, hyperthyroid, intestinal atony or obstruction, myasthenia gravis, prostatic hypertrophy, respiratory problems, tachycardia, ulcerative colitis, urinary retention

**Interactions**
Mantadine, antidiarrheals, antihistamines, antimuscarinics, CNS depressants, cortisone, haloperidol, levodopa, meperidine, methylphenidate, orphenadrine, phenothiazines, primidone, procainamide, quinidine, tranquilizers, tricyclic antidepressants

## Dose

*Adult* 0.5–6 mg/day; therapy should be initiated with a low dose and increased gradually at 5 or 6 day intervals

*Peds* Lower dose than adult; individualized

## Forms

Injection, tablets

## Adverse Effects

Blurred vision, constipation, difficult urination, dizziness, dry mouth, mydriasis, sedation, toxic psychosis, vomiting, weakness

## Special Nursing Considerations and Patient Education

- Store in light-resistant container.
- Monitor for fine vermicular tongue movements (may indicate early tardive dyskinesia).
- Administer after meal to aid in reduction of stomach upset.
- When discontinued, decrease dose gradually.
- Offer hard candy (regular or sugar-free) to relieve dry mouth.
- Be aware that
  - IM, IV, and oral doses are the same.
  - medication is cumulative; has abuse potential.
- Teach patient to
  - avoid alcohol and other CNS depressants.
  - be cautious when driving or involved in potentially hazardous tasks.
  - avoid strenuous activity in hot weather to prevent heat stroke.
  - notify physician if having eye pain, taking antipsychotics, experiencing GI complications.

# Butabarbital Sodium

**Brand Name**
   Butisol

**Actions**
   Depresses sensory cortex; decreases motor activity; alters cerebellar function; produces drowsiness, sedation, and hypnosis. Onset evident in 5–30 minutes.

**Uses**
   Hypnotic, sedative

**Contraindications**
*Meds* Alcohol, CNS depressants
*Other* Hepatic dysfunction, porphyria. *Use with caution:* Acute or chronic pain; cardiovascular, hepatic or renal dysfunction; hypertension; hypoadrenalism; hypotension; narrow-angle glaucoma; respiratory distress

**Interactions**
   Analgesics; anticonvulsants; antidepressants; antihistamines; barbiturates; corticosteroids; digitalis; digitoxin; doxycycline; griseofulvin; hypnotics; isoniazid; MAO inhibitors; narcotics; oral anticoagulants, antidiabetics, or contraceptives; phenylbutazone; sedatives; tranquilizers

**Dose**
*Adult* Hypnotic: 50–100 mg hs PO; sedative: 15–30 mg tid–qid PO
*Peds* 6 mg/kg/day in 3 divided doses

**Forms**
   Capsules, elixir, extended-action tablets, tablets

## Adverse Effects
Bradycardia, diarrhea, dizziness, drowsiness, emotional problems, excitement, hypotension, nausea, respiratory depression, vomiting

## Special Nursing Considerations and Patient Education
- Protect elixir from light.
- Reduce dosage for elderly or debilitated patients because of possibility of increased sensitivity.
- When discontinued, decrease dosage gradually.
- Be aware that
  - medication induces hepatic microsomal enzymes, resulting in increased metabolism of many drugs
  - medication is addictive.
- Teach patient to
  - be cautious when driving or involved in potentially hazardous tasks.
  - be cautious during cold weather (medication may substantially decrease body temperature).
  - avoid alcohol and other CNS depressants.

# Calcitriol (Vitamin D₃)

**Brand Name**
Rocaltrol

**Actions**
Stimulates calcium transport

**Uses**
Hypocalcemia of chronic renal dialysis

**Contraindications**
*Meds* Magnesium-containing antacids, vitamin D
*Other* Children, hypercalcemia, vitamin D toxicity.
*Use with caution:* Renal stones.

**Interactions**
Barbiturates, cholestyramine, digitalis, phenytoin, thiazide diuretics

**Dose**
*Adult* Individualized; initial dose: 0.25 $\mu$g/day; increase by 0.25 $\mu$g/day q2-4weeks after serum calcium levels are determined; *maximum* dose: 0.5-1 $\mu$g/day

**Forms**
Capsules

**Adverse Effects**
Bone or muscle pain, constipation, dry mouth, headache, nausea, somnolence, vomiting, weakness

**Special Nursing Considerations and Patient Education**
- Monitor serum calcium level.
- Offer hard candy (regular or sugar-free) to relieve dry mouth.
- Teach patient
  - to notify physician before taking any nonprescription drugs.
  - to adhere to prescribed increased-calcium diet.
  - that medication may cause metallic taste.

# Carbamazepine

**Brand Name**
Tegretol

**Actions**
Analgesic, anticonvulsant

**Uses**
Glossopharyngeal or trigeminal neuralgia; grand mal, mixed, or partial seizures

**Contraindications**
*Meds* MAO inhibitors
*Other* Bone-marrow depression, hypersensitivity to tricyclic antidepressants. *Use with caution:* Cardiovascular, hepatic, or renal dysfunction; increased intraocular pressure

**Interactions**
Doxycycline, oral anticoagulants or contraceptives, troleandomycin

**Dose**
*Adult* Initial dose: 200 mg/day; increase by 200 mg/day until best response is obtained; *maximum* recommended dose: 1,200 mg/day (up to 1,600 mg/day has been used in rare instances)
*Peds* 10–20 mg/kg/day

**Forms**
Tablets

**Adverse Effects**
Blood dyscrasias, confusion, congestive heart failure, dizziness, drowsiness, headache, leg cramps, nausea, unsteadiness, urinary retention, vomiting

## Special Nursing Considerations and Patient Education

- Monitor blood results (for dyscrasias), I&O, vital signs.
- When discontinued, decrease dosage gradually.
- If patient has tic douloureux, help identify behaviors that seem to provoke attacks.
- Administer with food to avoid GI upset.
- Teach patient to
  - be cautious when driving or involved in potentially hazardous tasks.
  - notify physician for fever, purpuric hemorrhage, sore throat, oral ulcers.

# Carisoprodol

**Brand Name**
Soma

**Actions**
Skeletal muscle relaxant; stops interneuronal activity in descending reticular formation. Onset evident in 30–60 minutes.

**Uses**
Acute painful musculoskeletal conditions

**Contraindications**
*Meds* Alcohol; allergic reactions to carisoprodol or related compounds such as meprobamate, mebutamate, or tybamate; CNS depressants
*Other* Acute intermittent porphyria, children under 12, idiosyncratic reaction to carisoprodol or other carbamates. *Use with caution:* Cerebral palsy, hepatic or renal dysfunction

**Interactions**
Anticonvulsants, antidepressants, antihistamines, barbiturates, hypnotics, MAO inhibitors, narcotics, phenothiazines, sedatives, tranquilizers

**Dose**
*Adult* 350 mg qid

**Forms**
Capsules, tablets

**Adverse Effects**
Ataxia, drowsiness, epigastric distress, erythema, headache, hiccoughs, nausea, orthostatic hypotension, tachycardia, tremors, vertigo, vomiting, weakness

## Special Nursing Considerations and Patient Education
- Administer with food or meals if GI upset occurs.
- Be aware that
  - dependence or tolerance can develop.
- Teach patient to
  - be cautious when driving or involved in potentially hazardous tasks.
  - avoid alcohol and other CNS depressants.
  - notify physician for dyspnea, fever, skin rash, visual disturbances.

# Carmustine (BCNU)

**Brand Name**
BiCNU

**Actions**
Antineoplastic; alkylating action on DNA/RNA

**Uses**
Brain tumors, combination therapy for Hodgkin's disease and non-Hodgkin's lymphomas, multiple myeloma (with prednisone)

**Contraindications**
*Meds* Smallpox vaccination
*Other* Decreased erythrocyte, leukocyte, and/or thrombocyte counts. *Use with caution:* Infection, renal dysfunction

**Interactions**
Hepatotoxics, myelosuppressives, nephrotoxics

**Dose**
*Adult* 150–200 mg/m², repeated in 6 weeks; may be given as single dose or divided in half and given on 2 successive days

**Forms**
Powder (for injection)

**Adverse Effects**
Diarrhea, hepatic toxicity, leukopenia, nausea, thrombocytopenia, vomiting

**Special Nursing Considerations
and Patient Education**
- Discard vials with oil films or powder liquefaction.
- Monitor for signs of hepatic toxicity (e.g., jaundice, pruritus) and renal insufficiency (e.g., dysuria, hematuria).
- Monitor temperature: elevation requires attention.
- Administer antiemetic prior to injection to help diminish or prevent nausea and vomiting.
- Administer over a 1- to 2-hour time span.
- Be aware that
  - burning, pain, and dizziness can occur during injection.
  - medication is cumulative.
- Teach patient
  - to notify physician of fever, signs of infection, sore throat.
  - precautions to take if CBC or platelet count falls (see Appendix C).
  - to maintain good hydration (approximately 10 to 12 glasses of fluid each day).

# Cephalexin

**Brand Name**
Keflex

**Actions**
Antibiotic (cephalosporin); impedes synthesis of mucopeptide cell walls

**Uses**
Infections of respiratory tract, skin and soft tissue, urinary tract

**Contraindications**
Hypersensitivity to cephalosporin antibiotics.
*Use with caution:* Allergy to penicillin, renal dysfunction

**Interactions**
Concomitant use with nephrotoxic agent (aminoglycosides) increases probability of nephrotoxicity; probenecid

**Dose**
*Adult*  250–500 mg q6h
*Peds*  Over 1 month of age: 25–50 mg/kg/day in 4 divided doses

**Forms**
Capsules, pediatric drops, suspension, tablets

**Adverse Effects**
Blood dyscrasias, diarrhea, dizziness, drowsiness, dyspepsia, headache, nausea, pseudomembranous colitis, urticaria, vomiting

## Special Nursing Considerations and Patient Education

- Refrigerate solutions and discard unused portion after 2 weeks.
- Monitor for nonsusceptible microbe overgrowth.
- Use Clinitest or Tes-Tape to test urine for sugar.
- Discontinue if diarrhea or rash occurs.
- Be aware that
  - sensitivity to penicillin may occur.
  - medication may cause false-positive Coombs' test and glycosuria.
- Teach patient to
  - complete full course of therapy.

# Chloral Hydrate

**Brand Name**
  Noctec

**Actions**
  Hypnotic, sedative. Onset evident in 30–60 minutes.

**Uses**
  Delirium tremens, hypnotic, sedative, withdrawal from barbiturates or narcotics

**Contraindications**
*Meds*  Alcohol, CNS depressants
*Other*  Cardiac, hepatic, or renal dysfunction; gastric ulcer; gastritis. *Use with caution:* Colitis, depression, drug abusers, proctitis

**Interactions**
  Antihistamines, barbiturates, furosemide, hypnotics, MAO inhibitors, narcotics, oral anticoagulants, phenothiazines, sedatives, tranquilizers, tricyclic antidepressants

**Dose**
*Adult*  PO: Hypnotic: 0.5–1 gm; sedative: 250 mg tid
*Peds*  PO: Hypnotic: 50 mg/kg; *maximum* dose: 1 gm; sedative: 25 mg/kg/day in 3–4 divided doses

**Forms**
  Capsules, elixir, suppository, syrup

**Adverse Effects**
  Confusion, dizziness, drowsiness, gastritis, hallucinations, headache, nausea, paradoxical behavior, peculiar taste, vomiting

## Special Nursing Considerations and Patient Education

- Refrigerate suppositories.
- Use caution when administering to patients with suicidal potential; ensure patient swallows dose.
- Mix liquid forms in a glass of fruit juice, ginger ale, or water.
- When used as a hypnotic, administer 15–30 minutes prior to hs.
- When discontinued, decrease dosage gradually.
- Be aware that
  - tolerance or addiction can develop.
- Teach patients to
  - be cautious when driving or involved in potentially hazardous tasks.
  - avoid alcohol and other CNS depressants.

# Chlorambucil

**Brand Name**
Leukeran

**Actions**
Antineoplastic, alkylating agent

**Uses**
Chronic lymphocyte leukemia, giant follicular lymphoma, Hodgkin's disease, reticulum cell carcinoma

**Contraindications**
Chemotherapy, radiation, smallpox vaccination.
*Use with caution:* Bone-marrow depression, history of gout or urate renal stones, infection, tumor cell infiltration into bone marrow

**Interactions**
Antigout agents

**Dose**
*Adult*  0.1–0.2 mg/kg/day for 3–6 weeks
*Peds*  0.1–0.2 mg/kg/day as a single or divided dose

**Forms**
Enteric-coated tablets

**Adverse Effects**
Anorexia, bone-marrow depression, cystitis, hyperuricemia, nausea, neurotoxicities, pulmonary fibrosis, vomiting

**Special Nursing Considerations
and Patient Education**
- Store medication in light-resistant containers.
- Decrease dose if sudden decrease in WBC occurs.
- Monitor blood studies weekly.
- Monitor I&O.
- Administer entire dose before breakfast or at hs to diminish nausea and vomiting.
- Be aware that
  - maximum daily dose with tumor infiltration of bone marrow is 0.1 mg/kg.
- Teach patient to
  - take medication exactly as prescribed.
  - notify physician of fever, signs of infections, sore throat.
  - maintain good hydration (approximately 10 to 12 glasses of fluid each day).
  - take precautions if CBC or platelet count falls (see Appendix C).

# Chlordiazepoxide HCl

**Brand Name**
Librium, A-poxide, Libritabs

**Actions**
Depression of limbic system of CNS and reticular formation of brainstem. Onset evident: PO 30–60 minutes; IM 15–30 minutes; IV 3–30 minutes.

**Uses**
Alcohol withdrawal, anticonvulsant, muscle relaxant, tranquilizer

**Contraindications**
*Meds* Alcohol, hypersensitivity to benzodiazepines
*Other:* Acute intermittent porphyria, acute narrow-angle glaucoma, children under 12, myasthenia gravis. *Use with caution:* Emphysema; hepatic, pulmonary, or renal dysfunction

**Interactions**
Anticonvulsants, antihistamines, barbiturates, cimetidine, CNS depressants, hypnotics, narcotics, oral anticoagulants, sedatives, tranquilizers

**Dose**
*Adult* PO: 5–25 mg bid–qid
*Peds* PO: Over 6 yr: 5 mg bid–qid

**Forms**
Capsules, injection, tablets

**Adverse Effects**
Ataxia, confusion, constipation, depression, dizziness, drowsiness, extrapyramidal symptoms, headache, lethargy

## Special Nursing Considerations and Patient Education

- Store medication in light-resistant containers.
- When discontinued, decrease dose gradually.
- When administering IM/IV, follow dispensing directions carefully. Use only diluent provided in package.
- Give IV dose slowly over at least 1 minute.
- Monitor I&O until drug dosage is stable.
- Monitor blood counts and liver function if therapy is continued over extended period of time.
- Be aware that
  - medication can be addictive and cumulative.
  - IM absorption is poor.
- Teach patient
  - to avoid prolonged exposure to sunlight since photosensitivity may occur.
  - that smoking may decrease effectiveness of medication.
  - to be cautious when driving or involved in potentially hazardous tasks.
  - to decrease caffeine intake because of its stimulant effects.
  - to notify physician for unusual bleeding, fever, sore throat.
  - to avoid alcohol and other CNS depressants.

# Chlorothiazide

**Brand Name**
  Diuril, Aldoclor, Diupress

**Actions**
  Diuretic; decreases reabsorption of chloride and
  sodium ions, which then leads to increased urinary
  output. Onset evident in 2 hours after oral
  ingestion.

**Uses**
  Antihypertensive, diuretic, edema

**Contraindications**
*Meds* Hypersensitivity to sulfonamide-derived
       medications, lithium
*Other* Anuria, hepatic or renal dysfunction. *Use
        with caution:* Diabetes, gout, hypercalcemia,
        hyperuricemia, lupus erythematosus,
        pancreatitis, postsympathectomy

**Interactions**
  Corticosteroids, corticotropin, oral antidiabetics

**Dose**
*Adult* PO: Antihypertensive: 500 mg bid; diuretic:
        500 mg–1 gm qd–bid
*Peds* PO: 20 mg/kg/day in 2 divided doses

**Forms**
  Oral suspension, sodium salt injection, syrup,
  tablets

**Adverse Effects**
  Anorexia, constipation, diarrhea, dizziness, muscle
  cramps, nausea, orthostatic hypotension,
  paresthesia, vomiting

## Special Nursing Considerations and Patient Education

- When used as a diuretic, administer in 1 dose in morning.
- Monitor blood pressure, I&O.
- Give patient diet containing potassium-rich foods (see Appendix F).
- Discontinue for electrolyte imbalance.
- Be aware that
  - IV form is not recommended for children.
- Teach patient
  - that medication may cause photosensitivity.
  - to be cautious when driving or involved in potentially hazardous tasks.
  - to be cautious during hot weather or strenuous exercise because of hypotensive effects.
  - that urine output will increase.
  - techniques to avoid orthostatic hypotension (e.g., getting up slowly).
  - to decrease coffee, tea, and high-salt foods in diet.
  - to decrease smoking.

# Chlorpheniramine Maleate

**Brand Name**

Chlor-Trimeton, Coricidin, Histaspan, AL-R

**Actions**

Antihistamine, antipruritic; hinders action of histamine. Onset evident in 15 minutes.

**Uses**

Allergic conjunctivitis, allergic and vasomotor rhinitis, blood/blood plasma allergies, pruritus, uncomplicated angioedema, urticaria

**Contraindications**

*Meds* Alcohol, CNS depressants, MAO inhibitors

*Other* Asthma, bladder-neck obstruction, narrow-angle glaucoma, neonates, premature infants, prostatic hypertrophy, respiratory tract infections, stenosing peptic ulcer. *Use with caution:* Cardiovascular dysfunction, hyperthyroidism, narrow-angle glaucoma, pyloroduodenal obstruction

**Interactions**

Anticholinergics, barbiturates, hypnotics, sedatives, tranquilizers, tricyclic antidepressants

**Dose**

*Adult* PO: 2–4 mg tid–qid

*Peds* PO: 2–6 yr: 1 mg tid–qid

6–12 yr: 1–2 mg tid–qid

**Forms**

Injection, sustained-release capsules, syrup, tablets

**Adverse Effects**

Anorexia, constipation, diarrhea, dizziness, drowsiness, dry mouth, euphoria, nausea, tinnitus, urticaria, vomiting

**Special Nursing Considerations
and Patient Education**
- Protect liquid forms from light.
- Keep out of reach of children.
- Do not crush sustained-release capsules.
- Administer medication with food or milk to reduce GI irritation.
- Teach patient
  - if allergic, to carry identification card that lists allergies.
  - to be cautious when driving or involved in potentially hazardous tasks.
  - to avoid alcohol and other CNS depressants.

# Chlorpheniramine Maleate/ Phenylephrine HCl/ Phenylpropanolamine HCl/ Phenyltoloxamine Citrate

**Brand Name**
Naldecon

**Actions**
Antihistamine, vasoconstrictor, vasopressor

**Uses**
Allergies, colds, orthostatic hypotension, upper respiratory problems

**Contraindications**
Diabetes, hypertension, hyperthyroidism, organic cardiac disease

**Interactions**
None

**Dose**
*Adult* 1 tablet tid or 5 cc q3-4h
*Peds* 2.5-10 cc q3-4h

**Forms**
Pediatric syrup or drops, syrup, tablets

**Adverse Effects**
Anxiety, drowsiness, GI upset

**Special Nursing Considerations
and Patient Education**
- Administer after meals to decrease irritation.
- Teach patient
  - to be cautious when driving or involved in potentially hazardous tasks.

# Chlorpheniramine Maleate/ Phenylpropanolamine

**Brand Name**
Novahistine

**Actions**
Antihistamine, decongestant

**Uses**
Allergic rhinitis, congestion of eustachian tube or nasal passages

**Contraindications**
*Meds* MAO inhibitors
*Other* Hyperthyroidism, severe coronary artery disease or hypertension. *Use with caution:* Cardiovascular disease, diabetes, hypertension, increased intraocular pressure, prostatic hypertrophy

**Interactions**
Alcohol, barbiturates, CNS depressants, tricyclic antidepressants

**Dose**
*Adult* 10 cc or 2 tablets q4h
*Peds* 2–5 yr: 2.5 cc q4h
6–12 yr: 5 cc or 1 tablet q4h

**Forms**
Liquid, tablets

**Adverse Effects**
Anxiety, CNS depression, dizziness, drowsiness, dry mouth, headache, hypertension, hypotension, insomnia, nausea, nervousness, respiratory difficulty, tension, vomiting

**Special Nursing Considerations
and Patient Education**
- Offer hard candy (regular or sugar-free) to relieve dry mouth.
- Teach patient to
  - change position slowly to decrease hypotension.
  - be cautious when driving or involved in potentially hazardous tasks.

# Chlorpromazine HCl

**Brand Name**
Thorazine

**Actions**
Antiemetic, antipsychotic, major tranquilizer.
Onset evident in 1–2 hours.

**Uses**
Acute intermittent porphyria, intractable
hiccoughs, nausea and vomiting, psychotic
disorders

**Contraindications**
*Meds* Alcohol, CNS depressants
*Other* Blood or bone-marrow disorders, children
under 6, coma. *Use with caution:* Cardiac,
hepatic, or respiratory dysfunction; epilepsy;
glaucoma; parkinsonism; peptic ulcer;
prostatic hypertrophy

**Interactions**
Antacids, antidiarrheals, atropine, guanethidine,
lithium, methyldopa, oral anticoagulants,
phenytoin, propranolol, trihexyphenidyl

**Dose**
*Adult* PO: 25 mg–1 gm in divided doses
*Peds* PO: 2 mg/kg/day in 4–6 divided doses

**Forms**
Capsules, injection, liquid, suppository, syrup,
tablets

**Adverse Effects**
Blood dyscrasias, constipation, dry mouth,
extrapyramidal symptoms, hypothermia, jaundice,

orthostatic hypotension, sedation, urinary
retention, weight gain

## Special Nursing Considerations and Patient Education

- Store medication in light-resistant container.
- Inject IM dose deeply; maximum of 1 cc per site; massage injection site.
- When discontinued, decrease dosage gradually.
- Monitor blood pressure, fecal and urinary output, fluid intake.
- Monitor for fine vermicular tongue movements (may indicate early tardive dyskinesia).
- Offer hard candy (regular or sugar-free) to relieve dry mouth.
- Use caution when administering to a patient with suicidal potential; ensure patient swallows dose.
- Teach patient
  - to be cautious when driving or involved in potentially hazardous tasks.
  - to take precautions during hot weather or strenuous exercise because of hypotensive effects.
  - to notify physician for bleeding, impaired vision, jaundice, rash, sore throat, tremors, weakness.
  - to remain recumbent for ½ hour following parenteral dosage of medication.
  - that medication may color urine brown, pink, or red.

# Chlorpropamide

**Brand Name**

Diabinese

**Actions**

Antidiabetic, hypoglycemic; stimulates secretion of insulin from pancreas

**Uses**

Diabetes (adult onset or noninsulin dependent)

**Contraindications**

*Meds*  Alcohol

Other  Diabetes associated with acidosis, infection, surgery, major trauma; endocrine, hepatic, or renal dysfunction; insulin-dependent or juvenile diabetes. *Use with caution:* Peptic ulcer, porphyria, thyroid dysfunction

**Interactions**

Clofibrate, corticosteroids, digitoxin, insulin, MAO inhibitors, nonsteroidal anti-inflammatory agents, oral contraceptives, oxyphenbutazone, phenylbutazone, probenecid, salicylates, sulfonamides, thiazide diuretics

**Dose**

*Adult*  100–250 mg/day

**Forms**

Tablets

**Adverse Effects**

Diarrhea, GI problems, hepatic toxicities, hypoglycemia, photosensitivity

**Special Nursing Considerations
and Patient Education**
- Monitor exercise, I&O, weight.
- Teach patient to
  - follow prescribed diet.
  - recognize signs of hyper- and hypoglycemia (see Appendix B).
  - take medication every day, except on professional advice.
  - avoid alcohol because of potential alcohol intolerance.

# Chlorprothixene

**Brand Name**
Taractan

**Actions**
Antipsychotic; depresses brainstem

**Uses**
Depression, neurosis, schizophrenia, withdrawal from alcohol

**Contraindications**
*Meds* Alcohol, CNS depressants
*Other* Coma. *Use with caution:* Cardiovascular disease, hepatic or respiratory dysfunction, parkinsonism, peptic ulcer, urinary retention

**Interactions**
Antacids, antidiarrheals, atropine, guanethidine, lithium, oral anticoagulants, phenytoin, propranolol, trihexyphenidyl

**Dose**
*Adult* PO: 25–50 mg tid–qid
*Peds* PO: 6–12 yr: 10–25 mg tid–qid

**Forms**
Concentrate, injection, tablets

**Adverse Effects**
Dizziness, drowsiness, dry mouth, extrapyramidal symptoms, lethargy, orthostatic hypotension, tachycardia

## Special Nursing Considerations
## and Patient Education
- Mix concentrate with liquids to mask taste.
- When discontinued, decrease dosage gradually.
- Monitor for fine vermicular tongue movements (may indicate early tardive dyskinesia).
- Offer hard candy (regular or sugar-free) to relieve dry mouth.
- Be aware that
  - IM form is not recommended for children.
- Teach patient
  - that medication may cause photosensitivity.
  - to be cautious when driving or involved in potentially hazardous tasks.
  - to notify physician for unusual bleeding, jaundice, rash, sore throat, tremors, vision impairment, weakness.
  - to change position slowly to avoid orthostatic hypotension.

# Chlortetracycline HCl

**Brand Name**
Aureomycin

**Actions**
Antiamebic, antibacterial, antibiotic, anti-infective, antirickettsial; hinders formation of essential proteins in bacteria

**Uses**
Superficial ocular and dermatologic infections

**Contraindications**
Hypersensitivity

**Interactions**
None

**Use**
Topical: apply tid
Ophthalmic ointment: apply small amount q3-4h

**Forms**
Dermatologic and ophthalmic ointment

**Adverse Effects**
Photosensitivity, superinfection (with prolonged use)

**Special Nursing Considerations
and Patient Education**
- Do not contaminate tip of ointment tube by
  touching eye.
- Teach patient that
  - ophthalmic ointment may cause temporary
    blurring of vision or stinging following
    administration.

# Chlorthalidone

**Brand Name**
   Hygroton, Regroton

**Actions**
   Diuretic; hinders reabsorption in tubules. Onset
   evident in 2 hours.

**Uses**
   Antihypertensive, diuretic, edema

**Contraindications**
*Meds*  Hypersensitivity to thiazides or sulfonamides
*Other*  Anuria, renal decompensation. *Use with
         caution:* Diabetes, gout, hypercalcemia,
         hyperuricemia, lupus erythematosus,
         pancreatitis, postsympathectomy

**Interactions**
   None

**Dose**
*Adult*  50–100 mg/day
*Peds*  3 mg/kg 3x/week

**Forms**
   Tablets

**Adverse Effects**
   Anorexia, constipation, diarrhea, dizziness,
   hypotension, light-headedness, muscle cramps,
   nausea, paresthesia, vomiting

**Special Nursing Considerations
and Patient Education**
- Administer whole dose in morning with breakfast.
- Teach patient to
  - be cautious during hot weather or strenuous exercise, because of possibility of electrolyte imbalance.
  - ingest foods rich in potassium (see Appendix F).
  - avoid licorice.
  - notify physician for unusual bruising, signs of electrolyte imbalance, fever, rash, sore throat, tingling, tremors.

# Chlorzoxazone

**Brand Name**
  Parafon Forte, Paraflex

**Actions**
  Skeletal muscle relaxant; hinders multisynaptic
  reflex arcs in subcortical brain and spinal cord.
  Onset evident in 1 hour.

**Uses**
  Adjunct in acute painful musculoskeletal
  conditions

**Contraindications**
  Alcohol, CNS depressants. *Use with caution:*
  Hepatic or renal dysfunction, history of or known
  allergies to muscle relaxants

**Interactions**
  Antihistamines, barbiturates, hypnotics, sedatives,
  tranquilizers

**Dose**
*Adult*  500–750 mg tid-qid
*Peds*  Based on age and weight: 125–500 mg tid-qid

**Forms**
  Tablets

**Adverse Effects**
  Angioneurotic edema, constipation, diarrhea,
  dizziness, drowsiness, dyspepsia, ecchymosis,
  headache, hepatic dysfunction, malaise, nausea,
  petechiae, tarry stools, vertigo, vomiting

**Special Nursing Considerations and
Patient Education**
- Protect medication from light.
- Crush tablets for easier administration.
- Teach patient
  - that medication may color urine pink or red.
  - to be cautious when driving or involved in
    potentially hazardous tasks.
  - to avoid alcohol and other CNS depressants.

# Cholestyramine

**Brand Name**
Questran

**Actions**
Antilipemic; increases oxidation of cholesterol into bile acids

**Uses**
Adjunct therapy in management of elevated cholesterol levels, pruritus caused by partial biliary obstruction

**Contraindications**
Complete biliary obstruction

**Interactions**
Digitalis, iron preparations, oral antibiotics or anticoagulants, phenylbutazone, thyroid hormones

**Dose**
*Adult* 4 gm tid–qid
*Peds* Over 6 yr: 80 mg/kg tid

**Forms**
Powder

**Adverse Effects**
Anorexia; bleeding; bloating; constipation; diarrhea; fecal impaction; hyperchloremic acidosis; malabsorption of vitamins A,D,E,K; nausea

## Special Nursing Considerations
## and Patient Education
- Administer all other medications 1–4 hours before or after this medication.
- Teach patient
  - to follow prescribed diet and to include increased fluids and roughage.
  - that medication may cause burnt odor in urine and/or bad taste in mouth.
  - to use a stool softener to help ease constipation.
  - never take medication in dry form; mix slowly with liquids.
  - place powder on top of 4–6 ounces of liquid and twirl glass slowly for several minutes. After drinking the solution, refill glass with liquid and drink this also.

# Cimetidine

**Brand Name**
Tagamet

**Actions**
Histamine antagonist. Onset of ulcer healing evident in 2 weeks after initiation of therapy.

**Uses**
Duodenal or gastric ulcer, hypersecretory disorders

**Contraindications**
Children under 16. *Use with caution:* Organic brain syndrome, renal dysfunction

**Actions**
Antacids, coumarin anticoagulants

**Dose**
*Adult* PO: 300 mg qid

**Forms**
Injection, liquid, tablets

**Adverse Effects**
Diarrhea, dizziness, gynecomastia, muscle pain, rash

**Special Nursing Considerations
and Patient Education**
- Be aware that
  - treatment should only last for 8 weeks unless
    specifically directed otherwise by physician.
- Teach patient to
  - be cautious when driving or involved in
    potentially hazardous tasks.

# Cisplatin

**Brand Name**
  Platinol

**Actions**
  Antineoplastic

**Uses**
  Ovarian or testicular carcinomas.

**Contraindications**
*Meds* Smallpox vaccination
*Other* Bone-marrow suppression, hearing or renal
  dysfunction, hypersensitivity to platinum
  compounds. *Use with caution:* Gout, history of
  urate renal stones, infection, radiation

**Interactions**
  Aminoglycosides, antigout medications,
  nephrotoxics, ototoxics

**Dose**
*Adult* Given in combination with other drugs.
  Ovarian ca: 100 mg/m² q4weeks; testicular ca:
  20 mg/m²/day, for 5 days q3weeks

**Forms**
  Powder (for injection)

**Adverse Effects**
  Alopecia, anaphylactic reaction, anorexia,
  bleeding, edema, hearing difficulties, leukopenia,
  nausea, nephrotoxicity, ototoxicity, peripheral
  neuropathy, thrombocytopenia, urinary difficulties,
  vomiting

**Special Nursing Considerations
and Patient Education**
- Store vials in refrigerator.
- Prior to administration, hydrate patient with 1–2 liters of fluid via IV infusion over 8–12 hours.
- Check that audiometry was done prior to initiating therapy and before subsequent doses.
- Hold repeat doses unless serum creatinine is 1.5 mg/100 cc and/or BUN is 25 mg/100 cc, platelet count is at least 100,000/mm³, WBC is at least 4,000/mm³, and there are no abnormalities noted on audiogram.
- Monitor renal function.
- Be aware that
  - medication is cumulative.
- Teach patient to
  - maintain good hydration (approximately 10 to 12 glasses of fluid each day).
  - notify physician for bleeding, fever, hearing difficulties, infection, sore throat, urinary problems.
  - take precautions if CBC or platelet count falls (see Appendix C).

# Clonazepam

**Brand Name**
Clonopin

**Actions**
Anticonvulsant; affects minor motor seizures (amplitude, duration, frequency, spread of discharge)

**Uses**
Akinesia, Lennox-Gastat syndrome, myoclonic seizures

**Contraindications**
*Meds* Alcohol, antihistamines, barbiturates, CNS depressants, hypnotics, narcotics, phenothiazines, sedatives, tricyclic antidepressants
*Other* Acute narrow-angle glaucoma, hepatic dysfunction

**Interactions**
Phenobarbital, phenytoin

**Dose**
*Adult* Initial dose: 1.5 mg/day in 3 divided doses; dosage may be increased in increments of 0.5–1 mg q3days until seizures are controlled; *maximum* dose: 20 mg/day
*Peds* Up to 10 yr: 0.01–0.03 mg/kg/day in 2–3 divided doses; over 10 yr: same as adult

**Forms**
Tablets

**Adverse Effects**

Anemia, anorexia, aphonia, ataxia, behavior problems, bruising, chest congestion, choreiform movements, confusion, depression, drowsiness, dry mouth, encopresis, hallucinations, palpitations, psychoses, rhinorrhea

**Special Nursing Considerations and Patient Education**

- Use caution when administering to patients with suicidal potential, ensure patient swallows dose.
- Monitor seizure activity.
- Offer hard candy (regular or sugar-free) to relieve dry mouth.
- Be aware that
  - medication can cause dependence; when discontinued, decrease dosage gradually.
- Teach patient
  - to be cautious when driving or involved in potentially hazardous tasks.
  - that medication may cause an increase in salivation or a feeling of coated tongue.
  - to carry some type of Medic Alert card or bracelet.

# Clonidine HCl

**Brand Name**
Catapres, Combipres

**Actions**
Vasodilator; decreases ability of sympathetic nervous system to maintain blood vessel constriction. Onset evident in 30–60 minutes.

**Uses**
Antihypertensive, withdrawal from narcotics (investigational use)

**Contraindications**
*Meds* Alcohol, CNS depressants
*Other* Children, diabetes. *Use with caution:* Cardiovascular dysfunction, chronic renal failure

**Interactions**
Tolazoline, tricyclic antidepressants

**Dose**
*Adult* Initial dose: 0.1 mg bid; *maximum* effective dose: 2.4 mg/day

**Forms**
Tablets

**Adverse Effects**
Bradycardia, congestive heart failure, constipation, depression, drowsiness, dry mouth, fatigue, headache, insomnia, nausea, orthostatic hypotension, vivid dreams, vomiting, weight gain

## Special Nursing Considerations and Patient Education

- Take blood pressure prior to administering medication.
- Monitor behavioral changes, blood pressure, I&O, neurologic status, weight.
- When discontinued, decrease dosage gradually over 2–4 days; give last dose at hs.
- Offer hard candy (regular or sugar-free) to relieve dry mouth.
- Be aware that
  - tolerance can develop.
  - if discontinued abruptly, a rapid increase in blood pressure is possible.
- Teach patient
  - to be cautious when driving or involved in potentially hazardous tasks.
  - about the possibility of weight gain and individually prescribed weight-control diet.
  - to monitor blood pressure for a month following discontinuation of treatment.
  - to change position slowly to avoid orthostatic hypotension.

# Cloxacillin Sodium

**Brand Name**
  Tegopen

**Actions**
  Antibiotic; hinders production of cell walls during
  replication

**Uses**
  Infections with penicillinase-producing
  staphylococci

**Contraindications**
  Allergy to penicillin. *Use with caution:* Allergy to
  cephalosporins, history of general allergies, renal
  dysfunction

**Interactions**
  Chloramphenicol, erythromycin, probenecid,
  tetracycline

**Dose**
  *Adult*  250–500 mg q6h
  *Peds*  Up to 20 kg: 50–100 mg/kg/day in divided
    doses q6h

**Forms**
  Capsules, solution

**Adverse Effects**
  Diarrhea, nausea, vomiting, wheezing

**Special Nursing Considerations
and Patient Education**
- Refrigerate solution and use within 2 weeks.
- Monitor patient for allergic reactions to medication.
- Administer medication 1 hour before or 2 hours after meals.

# Codeine Phosphate, Sulfate

**Brand Name**
  Methylmorphine

**Actions**
  Narcotic; acts on CNS and GI tract. Onset evident in 15–30 minutes.

**Uses**
  Analgesic, antitussive

**Contraindications**
*Meds*  Alcohol, hypersensitivity to narcotics, MAO inhibitors
*Other*  Bronchial asthma, head injuries, respiratory depression. *Use with caution:* Addison's disease, cardiac dysrhythmias, chronic ulcerative colitis, gallbladder, hepatic or renal dysfunction, prostatic hypertrophy, urethral stricture

**Interactions**
  Anticholinergics, antidepressants, antihistamines, general anesthetics, hypnotics, MAO inhibitors, phenothiazines, sedatives, skeletal muscle relaxants, tranquilizers, tricyclic antidepressants

**Dose**
*Adult*  PO: Analgesic: 15–60 mg qid; antitussive: 8–20 mg q3–4h
*Peds*  PO: Analgesic: 3 mg/kg/day in 6 divided doses antitussive: 1–1.5 mg/day in 6 divided doses

**Forms**
  Phosphate injection, syrup, tablets

**Adverse Effects**
  Constipation, dizziness, drowsiness, excitement, restlessness

**Special Nursing Considerations
and Patient Education**
- Store medication in light-resistant container.
- When discontinued, decrease dosage gradually.
- Be aware that
  - usual preparations are combinations of 2 or
    more drugs.
  - medication can habit forming.
- Teach patient
  - to be cautious when driving or involved in
    potentially hazardous tasks.

# Cromolyn Sodium

**Brand Name**
Intal

**Actions**
Antiasthmatic; hinders release of histamine. Onset evident in 4 weeks.

**Uses**
Adjunct for bronchial asthma

**Contraindications**
Acute asthma attack, children under 5, eosinophilic pneumonia, status asthmaticus. *Use with caution:* Hepatic or renal dysfunction, lactose hypersensitivity

**Interactions**
Cortisone-like drugs

**Dose**
*Adult* Contents of 1 capsule qid at regular intervals
*Peds* Over 5 yr: same as adult

**Forms**
Capsules (for inhalation)

**Adverse Effects**
Angioedema, bronchospasm, cough, dermatitis, hoarseness, nasal congestion, nausea, urticaria

**Special Nursing Considerations
and Patient Education**
- Store medication away from heat and moisture.
- Use Spinhaler turbo-inhaler with capsules.
- Do not use for acute attacks.
- When discontinued, decrease dose gradually.
- Teach patient
  - NOT to swallow the capsules.
  - not to exhale into the inhaler.
  - to avoid all allergens.
  - after removing inhaler, to hold breath for a few
    seconds.
  - to gargle and rinse mouth after each use.

# Cyclandelate

**Brand Name**
Cyclospasmol

**Actions**
Peripheral vasodilator, spasmolytic; relaxes smooth vascular muscle. Onset evident in 15 minutes.

**Uses**
Adjunct for arteriosclerosis obliterans, intermittent claudication, ischemic cerebral vascular disease, nocturnal leg cramps, Raynaud's disease, thrombophlebitis

**Contraindications**
None. *Use with caution:* Active bleeding or tendency to bleed, cerebrovascular dysfunction, CVA, glaucoma, MI, obliterative coronary artery disease

**Interactions**
Tricyclic antidepressants

**Dose**
*Adult* 200–400 mg qid (ac and hs)

**Forms**
Capsules, tablets

**Adverse Effects**
Diaphoresis, dizziness, flushing, GI distress, headache, tachycardia, tingling of extremities, weakness

**Special Nursing Considerations
and Patient Education**
- Protect medication from heat and light.
- Administer with meals, immediately following meals, or use antacids to decrease GI distress.
- Be aware that
  - medication results in improvement over period of time.
- Teach patient to
  - decrease smoking.

# Cyclobenzaprine HCl

**Brand Name**
Flexeril

**Actions**
Central-acting muscle relaxant

**Uses**
Adjunct in acute, painful musculoskeletal
conditions

**Contraindications**
*Meds* Alcohol, CNS depressants, MAO inhibitors
*Other* Cardiac dysrhythmias, children under 15,
congestive heart failure, heart block,
hyperthyroidism, recovering MI. *Use with
caution:* History of urinary retention

**Interactions**
Anticholinergics, guanethidine

**Dose**
*Adult* 10 mg tid; not recommended for use longer
than 2–3 weeks

**Forms**
Tablets

**Adverse Effects**
Blurred vision, cardiac irregularities, dizziness,
drowsiness, dry mouth, dyspepsia, insomnia,
paresthesia, tachycardia, weakness

## Special Nursing Considerations and Patient Education

- Administer for 2–3 weeks only.
- When discontinued, decrease dosage gradually.
- Offer hard candy (regular or sugar-free) to relieve dry mouth.
- Teach patient to
  - be cautious when driving or involved in potentially hazardous tasks.

# Cytarabine

**Brand Name**
Cytosar-U

**Actions**
Antimetabolite, antineoplastic; hinders synthesis of deoxycytidine

**Uses**
Acute leukemia

**Contraindications**
Smallpox vaccination. *Use with caution:* History of gout, infection, myelosuppressive radiation, renal failure, tumor cell infiltration of bone marrow

**Interactions**
None

**Dose**
*Adult* IV: 2 mg/kg/day in a single dose for 10 days; infusion: 0.5 mg/kg/day
*Peds* Same as adult

**Forms**
Powder (for injection)

**Adverse Effects**
Anemia, anorexia, bone-marrow suppression, diarrhea, freckling, leukopenia, nausea, skin ulceration, stomatitis, thrombocytopenia, ulcers, vomiting

## Special Nursing Considerations and Patient Education

- Store unreconstituted drug in refrigerator. Once reconstituted, store at room temperature and use within 48 hours.
- Discard any solution if a haze is present.
- Monitor blood work and I&O daily.
- Teach patient to
  - notify physician for bleeding, fever, infection, sore throat.
  - maintain good hydration (approximately 10 to 12 glasses of fluid each day).
  - take precautions if CBC or platelet count falls (see Appendix C).

# Danazol

**Brand Name**
Danocrine

**Actions**
Antigonadotropin; hinders output of follicle-stimulating hormone and luteinizing hormone

**Uses**
Endometriosis, fibrocystic breast disease, hereditary angioedema

**Contraindications**
Cardiac, hepatic, or renal dysfunction; lactation; pregnancy; undiagnosed genital bleeding. *Use with caution:* Epilepsy, migraine

**Interactions**
Insulin, warfarin

**Dose**
*Adult* 400 mg bid for 3–6 months

**Forms**
Capsules

**Adverse Effects**
Androgenic effects (decreased breast size, deepening of the voice, flushing, hirsutism), nervousness, vaginitis

**Special Nursing Considerations
and Patient Education**
- Observe for fluid retention.
- Discontinue if pregnancy is suspected.
- Be aware that
  - nonhormonal contraceptive measures are recommended during therapy.
  - ovuiation begins 60–90 days after medication is discontinued.

# Demeclocycline HCl

## Brand Name
Declomycin

## Actions
Antiamebic, antibacterial, antibiotic, anti-infective, antirickettsial; hinders protein synthesis in select microorganisms. Onset evident in 2–5 days.

## Uses
Granuloma inguinale, lymphogranuloma, mycoplasms, ornithosis, psittacosis, rickettsial disease, spirochetal relapsing fever

## Contraindications
*Meds* Antacids, antidiarrheals, dairy products
*Other* Children under 9, renal dysfunction. *Use with caution:* Hepatic or renal dysfunction

## Interactions
Anticoagulants, iron and mineral preparations, methoxyflurane, sodium bicarbonate

## Dose
*Adult* 150 mg q6h or 300 mg q12h
*Peds* Over 9 yr: 3–6 mg/kg/day in 2–4 divided doses

## Forms
Capsules, tablets

## Adverse Effects
Diabetes insipidus syndrome, increased skin pigmentation, nausea, superinfections

**Special Nursing Considerations
and Patient Education**
- Store in light-resistant containers.
- Administer oral forms 1 hour before or 2 hours after meals.
- Monitor I&O if therapy is prolonged.
- Teach patient
  - that medication may cause photosensitivity.
  - to take entire course of treatment.

# Desipramine HCl

**Brand Name**
Norpramin, Pertofrane

**Actions**
Antidepressant. Onset evident in 1–2 weeks.

**Uses**
Endogenous or reactive depression

**Contraindications**
*Meds* Alcohol, MAO inhibitors
*Other* Children, narrow-angle glaucoma, recent MI.
*Use with caution:* Asthma, cardiac disease,
diabetes, epilepsy, hyperthyroid, bipolar
disorders, prostatic hypertrophy, psychoses

**Interactions**
Adrenergics, anticholinergics, antihistamines,
clonidine, ethchlorvynol, guanethidine, hypnotics,
narcotics, procainamide, quinidine, sedatives,
thyroid preparations, tranquilizers

**Dose**
*Adult* 25–50 mg tid; dosage above 300 mg/day not
recommended
*Peds* Adolescent: 25–100 mg/day

**Forms**
Capsules, tablets

**Adverse Effects**
Blurred vision, constipation, dizziness, drowsiness,
dry mouth, impaired urination

**Special Nursing Considerations
and Patient Education**
- Use caution when administering to a patient with suicidal potential; ensure patient swallows dose.
- Monitor blood pressure until dosage is regulated.
- Offer hard candy (regular or sugar-free) to relieve dry mouth.
- When discontinued, decrease dosage gradually.
- Teach patient
  - to change position slowly to avoid orthostatic hypotension.
  - that medication may cause photosensitivity and peculiar taste in mouth.
  - to be cautious when driving or involved in potentially hazardous tasks.
  - to refrain from taking other medications for 2 weeks following discontinuation of this medication.

# Deslanoside

**Brand Name**
  Cedilanid-D

**Actions**
  Cardiac glycoside. Onset evident in 10–30 minutes.

**Uses**
  Cardiac failure

**Contraindications**
  Heart block caused by digitalis; ventricular
  fibrillation, tachycardia. *Use with caution:* Acute
  MI, chronic constrictive pericarditis, hypokalemia,
  idiopathic hypertrophic subaortic stenosis,
  incomplete AV block, myxedema, renal dysfunction

**Interactions**
  Adrenergic agents, calcium, procainamide,
  propranolol, quinidine, thyroid preparations

**Dose**
*Adult*  IM/IV: *initial* dose, 1.2–1.6 mg; *maintenance*
    dose individualized; should be with oral
    digitalis preparations after 12 hr
*Peds*  IM/IV: *initial* dose 22 μl/kg; *maintenance* dose:
    Same as adult

**Forms**
  Injection

**Adverse Effects**
  Anorexia, diarrhea, drowsiness, fatigue, headache,
  nausea, restlessness, visual disturbances,
  vomiting, weakness

**Special Nursing Considerations
and Patient Education**
- Store medication in light-resistant containers.
- Medication is toxic; observe for signs of toxicity
  (e.g., anorexia, diarrhea, nausea, vomiting).
- With larger volumes of medication, inject at two
  different sites.
- Monitor cardiac status (EKG).
- Teach patient to
  - notify physician of anorexia, dysrhythmias,
    blurred vision, diarrhea, nausea, visual color
    disturbances.

# Desoxyribonuclease/Fibrinolysin

**Brand Name**
Elase

**Actions**
Topical enzyme

**Uses**
Circumcision, episiotomy, 2nd and 3rd degree burns, surgical wounds, ulcerative lesions

**Contraindications**
Hypersensitivity. *Use with caution:* Sensitivity to bovine origin materials

**Interactions**
None

**Dose**
*Adult* Apply bid-tid q6-10h
*Peds* Same as adult

**Forms**
Ointment, powder (for solution)

**Adverse Effects**
Angioneurotic edema, maculopapular or vesicular dermatitis, pruritus, urticaria

**Special Nursing Considerations
and Patient Education**
- Refrigerate ointment.
- Do not use reconstituted solutions after 24 hours.
- Monitor condition of wound.
- Use aseptic technique with wounds.

# Dexamethasone

**Brand Name**

Decadron, Dexone, Hexadrol

**Actions**

Anti-inflammatory, glucocorticoid. Onset evident in 24–48 hours.

**Uses**

Allergies, cerebral edema resulting from brain metastasis, inflammations

**Contraindications**

Active eye infection, peptic ulcer, or tuberculosis; systemic fungal infection. *Use with caution:* Diabetes, glaucoma, hypertension, hypothyroidism, myasthenia gravis, thrombophlebitis

**Interactions**

Barbiturates, coumarin anticoagulants, digitalis preparations, ephedrine, insulin, oral antidiabetics, phenytoin, rifampin

**Dose**

*Adult* PO: 0.5–9 mg/day
*Peds* PO: 0.2 mg/kg/day in divided doses

**Forms**

Aerosol inhaler or skin spray, elixir, cream, injection, liquid, ophthalmic ointment or solution, tablets

**Adverse Effects**

Dry nose, epistaxis, fluid and electrolyte disturbances, headache, hypertension, insomnia, retention of sodium

## Special Nursing Considerations and Patient Education
- Monitor height (children), weight.
- Give high-protein diet.
- Be aware that
  - medication may cause dependence; when discontinued, decrease dosage gradually.
- Teach patient to
  - stop/decrease smoking.
  - carry some type of Medic Alert card or bracelet.
  - notify physician of menstrual irregularities, muscle weakness, vertigo.
  - (diabetic patient) test urine for glucose at least daily.

# Dexbrompheniramine Maleate/ Pseudoephedrine Sulfate

**Brand Name**
Disophrol

**Actions**
Antihistamine, vasoconstrictor

**Uses**
Acute rhinitis, congestion of eustachian tube, perennial or seasonal allergies, rhinosinusitis

**Contraindications**
Children under 12, coronary artery disease, severe hypertension. *Use with caution:* Cardiovascular disease, diabetes, glaucoma, hyperthyroidism, prostatic hypertrophy

**Interactions**
Alcohol, CNS depressants

**Dose**
*Adult* 1 tablet qid

**Forms**
Tablets

**Adverse Effects**
Abdominal cramps, anorexia, anxiety, CNS stimulation, confusion, dizziness, headache, hypertension, nausea, palpitations, tachycardia, tension, vertigo, vomiting

**Special Nursing Considerations
and Patient Education**
- Teach patient to
  - be cautious when driving or involved in
    potentially hazardous tasks.

# Dexchlorpheniramine Maleate

**Brand Name**
Polaramine

**Actions**
Antihistamine; competitive antagonist to histamine

**Uses**
Allergies, angioedema, asthma, atopic and contact dermatitis, eczema, migraine headaches, pruritus ani or vulvae, rhinitis, urticaria

**Contraindications**
*Meds* MAO inhibitors
*Other* Lactation. *Use with caution:* Bladder-neck obstruction, cardiovascular disease, hypertension, hyperthyroid, narrow-angle glaucoma, prostatic hypertrophy, stenosing peptic ulcer

**Interactions**
Alcohol, CNS depressants, phenothiazines

**Dose**
*Adult* 2 mg tid–qid
*Peds* Infants: 0.5 mg tid–qid
Under 12 yr: 1 mg tid–qid

**Forms**
Sustained-release tablets, syrup, tablets

**Adverse Effects**
Anorexia, blurred vision, diaphoresis, difficult urination, dizziness, drowsiness, dry mouth, GI distress, headache, nervousness, tachycardia

**Special Nursing Considerations
and Patient Education**
- Do not crush sustained-release tablets.
- Offer hard candy (regular or sugar-free) to relieve dry mouth.
- Teach patient to
  - be cautious when driving or involved in potentially hazardous tasks.

# Dextroamphetamine Sulfate

**Brand Name**
Dexedrine

**Actions**
Anorexiant, cerebral stimulant, sympathomimetic.
Onset evident in 30–60 minutes.

**Uses**
Adjunct in treatment of obesity, minimal brain
dysfunction, narcolepsy

**Contraindications**
*Meds* MAO inhibitors
*Other* Agitated states, angina pectoris, arteriosclerosis, cardiovascular disease, diabetes,
history of drug abuse, hyperexcitability,
hypertension, hyperthyroidism, nephritis,
tension. *Use with caution:* Arteriosclerosis,
CVA, glaucoma; hypertension, psychoses

**Interactions**
Antihypertensives, insulin, tricyclic
antidepressants

**Dose**
*Adult* 2.5–10 mg qd–tid; narcolepsy: 5–60 mg/day
*Peds* 2–15 mg/day in 2–3 divided doses

**Forms**
Elixir, long-acting capsules, tablets

**Adverse Effects**
Anorexia, constipation, diarrhea, dizziness, dry
mouth, insomnia, nausea, nervousness,
restlessness

## Special Nursing Considerations and Patient Education

- Do not crush long-acting capsules.
- Monitor vital signs daily.
- Do not administer within 6 hours of hs.
- Offer hard candy (regular or sugar-free) to relieve dry mouth.
- Be aware that
  - medication may be habit forming; when discontinued, decrease dosage gradually.
- Teach patient
  - that medication may cause a metallic taste in mouth.
  - to avoid foods rich in tyramine (see Appendix F).
  - to be cautious when driving or involved in potentially hazardous tasks.
  - if hypertensive, to use caution during strenuous activities and to recognize signs of hypertensive difficulty (e.g., easy fatigue, headache, irritability, nervousness).

# Diazepam

## Brand Name
Valium

## Actions
Amnesic, anticonvulsant, hypnotic, sedative, skeletal muscle relaxant; depresses brainstem reticular formation and limbic system. Onset evident: PO 30–60 minutes; IM 15–30 minutes.

## Uses
Anxiety, diagnostic tests (e.g., cardioversion, esophagoscopy, gastroscopy), muscle spasms, preoperative, status epilepticus, tension, withdrawal from alcohol

## Contraindications
*Meds*  Alcohol, MAO inhibitors
*Other*  Acute alcohol intoxication, children (IM/IV: under 1 month; PO: under 6 months), coma, myasthenia gravis, narrow-angle glaucoma, shock. *Use with caution:* Depression; hepatic, pulmonary, or renal dysfunction; psychoses

## Interactions
Anticonvulsants, antidepressants, CNS depressants, hypnotics, narcotics, sedatives, tranquilizers

## Dose
*Adult*  PO: 2–10 mg bid–qid
*Peds*  PO: Over 6 months: 1–2.5 mg tid–qid
  Over 1 month: 1–2 mg q3–4h IM/IV

## Forms
Injection, tablets

## Adverse Effects

Dizziness, drowsiness, headache, hypotension, libido changes, nausea

## Special Nursing Considerations and Patient Education

- Do not allow IV to exceed 5 mg/minute.
- Use caution when administering to a patient with suicidal potential; ensure patient swallows dose.
- Discontinue for bruising, eye pain, fever, hemorrhage, sore throat.
- Be aware that
  - IM dose is absorbed erratically.
  - medication is cumulative and causes dependence; when discontinued, decrease dosage gradually.
  - medication may increase possibility of convulsions.
- Teach patient to
  - be cautious when driving or involved in potentially hazardous tasks.
  - decrease caffeine intake and smoking.
  - express feelings of anxiety openly.

# Diazoxide Injection

**Brand Name**
Hyperstat IV, Proglycem

**Actions**
Antihypertensive, antihypoglycemic; relaxes smooth peripheral vascular muscle. Onset evident in 5 minutes.

**Uses**
Dysmenorrhea, hypertensive emergency, hypoglycemia, premature labor

**Contraindications**
Thiazide hypersensitivity. *Use with caution:* Dialysis, impairment of cardiac or cerebral circulation

**Interactions**
Antidiabetics, hydralazine, methyldopa, nitrates, oral anticoagulants, reserpine, thiazide diuretics

**Dose**
*Adult*  Hypertension: 300 mg; hypoglycemia: 3–8 mg/kg in 2–3 divided doses
*Peds*  Infants: 8–15 mg/kg in 2–3 divided doses
Hypoglycemia: 3–8 mg/kg in 2–3 divided doses

**Forms**
Injection

**Adverse Effects**
Congestive heart failure, constipation, diarrhea, dysrhythmias, flushing, headache, nausea, orthostatic hypotension, palpitations, sodium and water retention

**Special Nursing Considerations
and Patient Education**
- Protect medication from freezing, heat, and light.
- Do not give IM or SC.
- Have patient remain recumbent for 30 minutes
  after administration. If also receiving furosemide,
  have patient remain recumbent for 8–20 hours.
- Inject rapidly (within 30 seconds).
- Monitor blood pressure q1min x 5, then at 5-minute
  intervals until stable, then hourly.
- Monitor I&O, weight.
- Teach patient that
  - medication may cause hirsutism on back,
    forehead, and limbs.

# Dicumarol

**Actions**

Anticoagulant; hinders synthesis of prothrombin. Onset evident in 24–72 hours.

**Uses**

Adjunctive treatment of coronary occlusion, atrial fibrillation associated with embolization, prophylaxis/treatment of pulmonary embolism or venous thrombosis

**Contraindications**

Continuous GI drainage, hemorrhagic conditions, subacute bacterial endocarditis. *Use with caution:* Congestive heart failure, diabetes, hepatic dysfunction, hypertension, occupational injury, vitamin C or K deficiency

**Interactions**

Anabolic steroids, barbiturates, broad spectrum antibiotics, chloral hydrate, chloramphenicol, cholestyramine, clofibrate, dextrothyroxine, disulfiram, estrogens, ethchlorvynol, glutethimide, oxyphenbutazone, phenylbutazone, salicylates, thyroid preparations, vitamin K

*Note:* Oral anticoagulants have greater potential for significant drug interactions than any other class of drugs.

**Dose**

Individualized; 200–300 mg/day

**Forms**

Capsules, tablets

**Adverse Effects**

Anorexia, dermatitis, diarrhea, fever, hemorrhage, nausea, vomiting

## Special Nursing Considerations and Patient Education

- When discontinued, decrease dosage gradually to prevent complications.
- Monitor prothrombin time daily during dosage adjustment, during maintenance, and at individually predetermined times.
- Teach patient to
  - not take other medications without notifying physician.
  - not change diet because of possible impact on response to medication.
  - use an electric razor to decrease danger of cutting self.
  - carry some type of Medic Alert card or bracelet.
  - use caution in hot weather because of impact on prothrombin time.
  - discontinue if evidence of blood in stools or urine and notify physician immediately.

# Digitoxin

**Brand Name**
Crystodigin, Purodigin, Unidigin

**Actions**
Cardiac glycoside; increases availability of calcium in heart muscle. Onset evident: PO 2-4 hours; IV 30 minutes–2 hours.

**Uses**
Dysrhythmias

**Contraindications**
Hepatic damage. *Use with caution:* Cardiac block, emphysema, hepatic or renal dysfunction, hypercalcemia, hypertrophic subaortic stenosis, hypokalemia, hypothyroidism, MI, myocarditis, myxedema, ventricular fibrillation

**Interactions**
Adrenergic agents, calcium, procainamide, propranolol, quinidine, thyroid preparations

**Dose**
*Adult*  PO: *Digitalizing* dose 1.2-1.6 mg;
        *maintenance* dose 0.05-0.3 mg/day
*Peds*  PO: 1 month–2 yr: *digitalizing* dose 0.04 mg/kg;
        over 2 yr: *digitalizing* dose 0.03 mg/kg;
        *maintenance* dose: 1/10 of digitalizing dose

**Forms**
Injection, tablets

**Adverse Effects**
Anorexia, confusion, diarrhea, disorientation, drowsiness, headache, increased salivation, irregular pulse, irritability, nausea, restlessness, visual disturbances, vomiting

## Special Nursing Considerations
## and Patient Education
- Take apical pulse prior to administration; if a change is noted, hold dose until you confer with physician. Monitor pulse as necessary per individual patient.
- Give IM dose deep into gluteal muscle, no more than 2 cc/site; massage site after injection.
- Notify physician of anorexia, dysrhythmias, blurred vision, diarrhea, irregular pulse, nausea, visual color disturbances.
- Protect medication from light.
- Be aware that
  - maintenance dose is usually given as a single dose in morning with meal.
- Teach patient
  - to decrease caffeine intake and smoking because of their stimulant effect.
  - of the possibility of taking medication for a lifetime.

# Digoxin

**Brand Name**
Lanoxin

**Actions**
Cardiotonic digitalis glycoside; increases force of myocardial contractions

**Uses**
Atrial fibrillation and flutter, congestive heart failure, paroxysmal atrial tachycardia

**Contraindications**
Complete atrio-ventricular block, ventricular tachycardia. *Use with caution:* Acute MI, emphysema, glomerulonephritis, hypercalcemia, idiopathic hypertrophic subaortic stenosis, ischemic cardiac or renal dysfunction, myocarditis, myxedema, pericarditis, increased serum potassium, rheumatic carditis, ventricular fibrillation

**Interactions**
Adrenergic agents, calcium, procainamide, propranolol, quinidine, thyroid preparations

**Dose**
*Adult* Digitalization; initial dose, PO: 2–3 mg; IV: 1–1.5 mg; IM: 1–2 mg; *maintenance* dose: 0.125–0.50 mg/day PO
*Peds* Digitalization; newborn: initial dose, 0.04–0.06 mg/kg PO; 1 month–2 yr: 0.06–0.08 mg/kg; over 2 yrs: 0.04–0.06 mg/kg; *maintenance* dose: usually 1/5–1/3 of digitalizing dose

**Forms**
Elixir, injection, pediatric elixir and injection, tablets

## Adverse Effects

Anorexia, diarrhea, drowsiness, fatigue, increased salivation, irregular pulse, nausea, pedal edema, vomiting, weakness; *in neonates:* prolongation of P-R interval, sinoatrial arrest, undue slowing of sinus rate

## Special Nursing Considerations and Patient Education

- Take apical/radial pulse for one minute prior to administration. Hold drug if rate is less than 60 for adults, 70 for pediatric patients. Identify individualized pulse monitoring guidelines.
- Inject IM dose into deep muscles; give no more than 2 cc at 1 site; massage site after administration.
- Protect medication from light.
- Monitor I&O; take weight daily.
- Be aware that
  - therapy with this medication is usually ongoing.
- Teach patient to
  - carry some type of Medic Alert card or bracelet.
  - notify physician of anorexia, dysrhythmias, blurred vision, changes in pulse rate or regularity, diarrhea, nausea, visual color disturbances.

# Dimenhydrinate

**Brand Name**
Dramamine

**Actions**
Antinauseant; decreases motion-caused stimulation of labyrinth structures. Onset evident in 30–60 minutes.

**Uses**
Dizziness, nausea, vertigo, vomiting associated with motion sickness

**Contraindications**
*Meds*  Alcohol, CNS depressants, MAO inhibitors, ototoxics
*Other*  Allergies to diphenhydramine or theophylline; infants, neonates. *Use with caution:* Bladder-neck or pyloroduodenal obstruction, cardiovascular dysfunction, history of reactions to antihistamines, hypertension, hyperthyroidism, narrow-angle glaucoma, prostatic hypertrophy, stenosing peptic ulcer

**Interactions**
Aminoglycosides, tricyclic antidepressants

**Dose**
*Adult*  PO: 50–100 mg q4h; parenteral: 50 mg prn
*Peds*  PO: Over 3 yr: 1.25 mg/kg qid

**Forms**
Injection, suppository, syrup, tablets

**Adverse Effects**
Blurred vision, dizziness, drowsiness, headache, nausea, palpitations

**Special Nursing Considerations
and Patient Education**
- Be aware that tolerance can develop.
- Administer 30 minutes prior to travel to prevent motion sickness.
- Teach patient to
  - be cautious when driving or involved in potentially hazardous tasks.

# Diphenhydramine HCl

**Brand Name**
   Benadryl, Benylin

**Actions**
   Antiemetic, antiparkinsonism, antivertigo,
   histamine antagonist, hypnotic. Onset evident in
   30 minutes.

**Uses**
   Allergic reactions (blood, blood plasma,
   conjunctivitis, rhinitis), angioedema, intractable
   insomnia, motion sickness, parkinsonism, pruritus,
   urticaria

**Contraindications**
*Meds* Alcohol, CNS depressants, MAO inhibitors
*Other* Acute asthma, lactation, narrow-angle
   glaucoma, urinary retention. *Use with caution:*
   Cardiovascular disease, hypertension, hyperthyroidism, prostatic hypertrophy, pyloroduodenal obstruction, stenosing peptic ulcer

**Interactions**
   Epinephrine, phenothiazines

**Dose**
*Adult* PO: 25–50 mg tid–qid
*Peds* PO: 5 mg/kg in 4 divided doses

**Forms**
   Capsules, elixir, injection

**Adverse Effects**
   Constipation, dizziness, drowsiness, epigastric
   distress, headache, hypotension, nausea,
   tachycardia, vomiting

## Special Nursing Considerations and Patient Education

- Administer IV dose slowly, with patient recumbent.
- Counsel patient to avoid alcohol.
- Monitor impact of medication on the blood pressure of patients with blood pressure dysfunction.
- Give drug with meals or milk to reduce GI upset.
- Protect medication from light.
- Teach patient
  - to be cautious when driving or involved in potentially hazardous tasks.
  - that medication may cause decreased tolerance to contact lenses because of atropine-like effects.

# Diphenoxylate HCl/ Atropine Sulfate

**Brand Name**
Lomotil

**Actions**
Antidiarrheal; slows intestinal motility

**Uses**
Colostomy, diarrhea, ileostomy

**Contraindications**
*Meds* MAO inhibitors
*Other* Children under 2, cirrhosis, colitis, diarrhea as
a result of poisoning, glaucoma, hepatic
disease, jaundice. *Use with caution:* Addison's
disease, cardiovascular instability, dehydration,
diarrhea (infection), gallbladder or hepatic
disease, hiatal hernia, hypertension, hyperthyroidism, hypothyroidism, intestinal atony,
myasthenia gravis, prostatic hypertrophy, renal
dysfunction, urethral stricture

**Interactions**
Alcohol, amantadine, atropine-like drugs,
barbiturates, CNS depressants, haloperidol,
hypnotics, narcotics, phenothiazines, sedatives,
tranquilizers, tricyclic antidepressants

**Dose**
*Adult* 5 mg tid–qid
*Peds* 2–12 yr: (liquid only) 0.3–0.4 mg/kg/day in
divided doses

**Forms**
Liquid, tablets

**Adverse Effects**
   Blurred vision, dizziness, dry mouth, euphoria,
   headache, nausea, pruritus, restlessness, sedation,
   tachycardia, vomiting

**Special Nursing Considerations
and Patient Education**
- Protect medication from direct light.
- Reduce dose as quickly as possible.
- Observe for abdominal distention.
- Hold dose if electrolyte imbalance or dehydration
  occurs.
- Offer hard candy (regular or sugar-free) to relieve
  dry mouth.
- Administer medication only as directed,
  particularly liquid form.
- Be aware that
  - dependence is possible; when discontinued,
    decrease dose gradually.
- Teach patient
  - to be cautious when driving or involved in
    potentially hazardous tasks.

# Disopyramide Phosphate

**Brand Name**

Norpace

**Actions**

Antidysrhythmic; decreases excitability of cardiac muscle. Onset evident in 3 minutes.

**Uses**

Prevention and control of premature ventricular contractions

**Contraindications**

Cardiogenic shock, congestive heart failure (unless accompanied by dysrhythmia and patient is digitalized), glaucoma, heart block, hyper- and hypokalemia, sick-sinus syndrome, urinary retention. *Use with caution:* Bradycardia-tachycardia syndrome, bundle branch block, hepatic or renal dysfunction, left ventricle dysfunction, myasthenia gravis, myocarditis, Q-T prolongation less than 25%, Wolff-Parkinson-White Syndrome

**Interactions**

Barbiturates, glutethimide, phenytoin, primidone, rifampin

**Dose**

*Adult*  400–800 mg/day in divided doses; *loading* dose: 300 mg then 150 mg q6h; *maintenance* dose: 100–200 mg q6h

*Peds*  Under 1 yr: 10–30 mg/kg/day; 1 to 4 yr: 10–20 mg/kg/day; 4 to 12 yr: 10–15 mg/kg/day; 12–18 yr: 6–15 mg/kg/day

**Forms**

Capsules

## Adverse Effects

Anorexia, chest pain, conduction disturbance, congestive heart failure, constipation, diarrhea, dizziness, dry mouth, edema, eye pain, fatigue, hypoglycemia, hypotension, nausea, syncope, urinary hesitancy and retention, weakness, weight gain

## Special Nursing Considerations and Patient Education

- Administer after EKG has been recorded and evaluated.
- Discontinue for widening of QRS complex.
- Monitor serum potassium levels (baseline and at predetermined intervals), vital signs, weight.
- Offer hard candy (regular or sugar-free) to relieve dry mouth.
- Teach patient
  - not to discontinue medication without notifying physician.
  - to be cautious when driving or involved in potentially hazardous tasks.

# Dobutamine HCl

**Brand Name**
Dobutrex

**Actions**
Cardiac stimulant, sympathomimetic. Onset evident in 1-2 minutes.

**Uses**
Cardiac decompensation

**Contraindications**
*Meds* Incompatible with alkaline solutions
*Other* Acute MI, children, idiopathic hypertrophic subaortic stenosis. *Use with caution:* Hypertension, severe aortic valve stenosis

**Interactions**
Anesthetics, beta blockers, MAO inhibitors, nitroprusside, oxytocics, tricyclic antidepressants

**Dose**
*Adult* 2.5-10 μg/kg of body weight/minute; *maximum* dose: 40 μg/kg of body weight/minute

**Forms**
Injection

**Adverse Effects**
Angina, headache, hypertension, nausea, palpitations, shortness of breath, tachycardia, ventricular ectopic activity

**Special Nursing Considerations
and Patient Education**
- Monitor blood pressure, EKG, I&O, pulmonary artery wedge pressure.
- Correct hypovolemia before treatment is instituted.
- Do not add sodium bicarbonate or other alkaline solutions to this drug.

# Docusate Sodium
## (formerly Dioctyl Sodium Sulfosuccinate)

**Brand Name**
Colace

**Actions**
Cathartic, stool softener; increases addition of fatty substances and water to fecal matter. Onset evident in 1–3 days.

**Uses**
Chronic constipation, painful anus and/or rectum, rectal impaction

**Contraindications**
*Meds* Mineral oil
*Other* Abdominal pain, intestinal obstruction, nausea, vomiting

**Interactions**
Danthron

**Dose**
*Adult* 50–200 mg/day
*Peds* Infants and children under 3 yr: 10–40 mg/day; 3–6 yr: 20–60 mg/day; 6–12 yr: 40–120 mg/day

**Forms**
Capsules, liquid, syrup

**Adverse Effects**
Excessive bowel activity, mild or transitory cramping

**Special Nursing Considerations
and Patient Education**
- Administer with fruit juices or milk to mask taste,
  if necessary.
- Be aware that
  - prolonged, frequent, or excessive use may result
    in laxative dependence and/or electrolyte
    imbalance.

# Dopamine HCl

**Brand Name**
Intropin

**Actions**
Vasopressor; stimulation of alpha, beta, and dopaminergic receptors

**Uses**
Correction of hemodynamic imbalances in shock syndrome

**Contraindications**
Children, pheochromocytoma, tachydysrhythmias, ventricular fibrillation. *Use with caution:* History of occlusive vascular disease

**Interactions**
Cyclopropane, halogenated hydrocarbons, MAO inhibitors, phenytoin, tricyclic antidepressants

**Dose**
*Adult* Infusion: 2–5 μg/kg of body weight/minute, increased until desired response is obtained

**Forms**
Injection

**Adverse Effects**
Angina, dyspnea, ectopic beats, headache, hypotension, nausea, palpitations, tachycardia, vasoconstriction, vomiting

low dose
causes vasodilation of renal
and mesenteric arteries.
allows for ↑ renal blood flow &
150 greater amt of urine & Na
excretion. Prevents kidney
failure 2° → shock.

**Special Nursing Considerations
and Patient Education**
- Correct hypovolemia before giving this medication.
- Monitor blood pressure, cardiac output, EKG, color
  and temperature of extremities, infusion rate,
  pulmonary artery wedge pressure, pulse, urinary
  output.
- Do not add sodium bicarbonate or other alkaline
  solutions to this drug.

Absorption given parenterally
onset- 2-4 min
duration- 5-10 min

# Doxepin HCl

**Brand Name**
   Sinequan, Adapin

**Actions**
   Tricyclic antidepressant; hinders reuptake of
   norepinephrine. Onset evident in 2–3 weeks.

**Uses**
   Anxiety, endogenous depression

**Contraindications**
*Meds*  Alcohol, MAO inhibitors
*Other*  Children under 12, narrow-angle glaucoma,
         recent MI, urinary retention. *Use with caution:*
         Cardiac dysfunction, diabetes, epilepsy,
         glaucoma, hyperthyroidism, prostatic
         hypertrophy

**Interactions**
   Anticholinergics, clonidine, estrogen,
   ethchlorvynol, guanethidine, hypnotics, levodopa,
   narcotics, procainamide, quinidine, sedatives,
   sympathomimetics, thyroid preparations,
   tranquilizers

**Dose**
*Adult*  10–50 mg tid; additional effectiveness is rarely
         obtained by exceeding 300 mg/day

**Forms**
   Capsules, oral solution

**Adverse Effects**
   Blurred vision, drowsiness, dry mouth,
   extrapyramidal symptoms, decreased libido,
   nausea, tinnitus, vomiting, weight gain

## Special Nursing Considerations and Patient Education

- Do not dilute concentrate with carbonated beverages.
- Use caution when administering to a patient with suicidal potential; ensure patient swallows dose.
- When discontinued, decrease dosage gradually.
- Offer hard candy (regular or sugar-free) to relieve dry mouth.
- Teach patient
  - to be cautious when driving or involved in potentially hazardous tasks.
  - that medication may cause a peculiar taste in mouth.
  - that it will take approximately 2–3 weeks before effect is felt.

# Doxycycline Hyclate

**Brand Name**
Vibramycin

**Actions**
Antiamebic, antibacterial, antibiotic, anti-infective, antirickettsial; hinders bacteria's formation of proteins

**Uses**
Granuloma inguinale, lymphogranuloma, mycoplasma, ornithosis, psittacosis, rickettsial disease, spirochetal relapsing fever

**Contraindications**
*Meds* Antacids, iron and mineral preparations
*Other* Children. *Use with caution:* History of hepatic or renal dysfunction, lupus erythematosus

**Interactions**
Barbiturates, carbamazepine, methoxyflurane, oral anticoagulants, penicillin, phenytoin, sodium bicarbonate

**Dose**
*Adult* PO: Initial dose: 200 mg in 2 divided doses; *maintenance* dose: 100 mg/day PO or IV infusion
*Peds* PO: 100 lbs or less: initial dose, 4.4 mg/kg in 2 divided doses; *maintenance* dose: 2.2–4.4 mg/kg/day in 2 divided doses

**Forms**
Calcium salt syrup, hyclate capsules or injection, monohydrate suspension

**Adverse Effects**

Diarrhea, dysphagia, jaundice, nausea, renal impairment, superinfections, teeth discoloration (children), vomiting

**Special Nursing Considerations and Patient Education**

- Protect medication from light.
- Monitor urinary output.
- Teach patient
  - to continue medication for 24–48 hours after temperature returns to normal.
  - *not* to consume dairy products 1 hour before or after each dose, as they affect action of the medication.
  - to take dose 1 or 2 hours after eating.
  - that medication may cause photosensitivity.

# Ephedrine HCl

**Brand Name**
Quadrinal

**Actions**
Bronchodilator, vasoconstrictor

**Uses**
Asthma, congestion, enuresis, hypotension, shock

**Contraindications**
Narrow-angle glaucoma, psychoneuroses. *Use with caution:* Angina, cardiovascular disease, diabetes, hypertension, hyperthyroidism, prostatic hypertrophy

**Interactions**
Beta-adrenergic blocking agents, digitalis, MAO inhibitors, sympathomimetics, tricyclic antidepressants

**Dose**
*Adult*  15–50 mg q3–4h
*Peds*  3 mg/kg/day in 4–6 divided doses

**Forms**
Capsules, solution, syrup

**Adverse Effects**
Anorexia, anxiety, chest pain, dysuria, headache, insomnia, mood changes, nausea, palpitations, vomiting

## Special Nursing Considerations and Patient Education

- Protect medication from heat and light.
- Monitor blood pressure and pulse.
- Be aware that
  - tolerance can develop.
- Teach patient to
  - avoid taking medication prior to bedtime because of side effect of insomnia.
  - notify physician for bladder problems, cardiac complaints, eye pain.

# Epinephrine

**Brand Name**
Adrenalin Chloride, Primatene Mist

**Actions**
Adrenergic, antiallergic, bronchodilator, hemostatic, sympathomimetic, vasopressor; stimulates adrenergic receptors. Onset evident in 3–10 minutes.

**Uses**
Cardiac arrest, glaucoma, hypersensitivity, mucosal congestion, uterine muscle relaxation

**Contraindications**
*Meds* Digitalis, hyaluronidase, protein hydrolysates
*Other* Cerebral arteriosclerosis, hypertension, hyperthyroidism, narrow-angle glaucoma, pulmonary edema, shock. *Use with caution:* Angina, asthma, cardiac disease, diabetes, emphysema, psychoneuroses

**Interactions**
Antihistamines, isoproterenol, MAO inhibitors, sympathomimetics, tricyclic antidepressants

**Dose**
*Adult* SC: 0.5–1.5 mg; 1–2 inhalations q4h; IV: 1 mg of 1:10,000 solution
*Peds* SC: 0.01 mg/kg

**Forms**
Injection, oil suspension, ophthalmic and topical solutions

## Adverse Effects

Anxiety, chest pain, dizziness, dry mouth, headache, nausea, nervousness, palpitations, restlessness, vomiting

## Special Nursing Considerations and Patient Education

- Administer IV slowly in low concentrations.
- Use a tuberculin syringe to ensure accuracy.
- Monitor blood pressure, pulse, and patient's overall response after each administration.
- Follow instructions for parenteral administration closely.
- Rotate injection sites.
- Be aware that
  - tolerance can develop.
  - blood glucose levels may be increased by this medication.
- Teach patient
  - that ophthalmic solution and nose drops may sting.
  - to rinse out mouth and throat with water after inhalation to avoid ingestion of residual drug.

# Ergotamine/Caffeine

**Brand Name**
Cafergot, Bellergal, Ergomar

**Actions**
Constriction of blood vessels in head. Onset evident in 30–60 minutes.

**Uses**
Cluster or migraine headaches

**Contraindications**
*Meds* Alcohol
*Other* Angina, arteriosclerosis, Buerger's disease, children, coronary artery disease, hypertension, lactation, malnutrition, peripheral vascular disease, pruritus, Raynaud's disease, renal dysfunction, sepsis, severe infection, thrombophlebitis

**Interactions**
Amphetamines

**Dose**
*Adult* PO: 2 mg stat; then 2 mg after 30 minutes to a *maximum* of 6 mg/day; dosage should not exceed 10 mg/week

**Forms**
Aerosol inhaler, sublingual tablets, tablets

**Adverse Effects**
Confusion, diarrhea, ergotism, insomnia, paresthesia, tachycardia

160

**Special Nursing Considerations
and Patient Education**
• Protect medication from heat and light.
• Teach patient
  – to rest in a dark room after taking medication.
  – to be cautious when driving or involved in
    potentially hazardous tasks.
  – not to increase dosage without discussing it
    with physician.
  – to notify physician for signs of ergotism (e.g,
    confusion, diarrhea, pulse irregularities, thirst,
    vomiting).

# Estrogens, Conjugated

**Brand Name**
Premarin

**Actions**
Similar to endogenous estrogen; synthesis of selected proteins and RNA

**Uses**
Breast or prostatic cancer palliation, dysfunctional uterine hemorrhage, hypogonadism (female), kraurosis or pruritus vulvae, postpartum breast engorgement, senile vaginitis, vasomotor symptoms of menopause, possible prevention of post menopausal osteoporosis

**Contraindications**
Estrogen-dependent neoplasia, pregnancy, thromboembolic disorders, undiagnosed vaginal bleeding. *Use with caution:* Asthma, cardiac or renal dysfunction, children, epilepsy, jaundice, metabolic bone disease, migraine headache

**Interactions**
Tricyclic antidepressants

**Dose**
Adult  PO: 0.3–1.25 mg/day; IV/IM: 25 mg q6–12 hrs; intravaginal: cream, 2–4 gm/day
*Peds*  Adolescent: Individualized: 5–10 mg

**Forms**
Cream, injection, tablets

**Adverse Effects**
Abdominal cramps, chloasma, chorea, headache, hirsutism, menstrual abnormalities, nausea, vaginal hemorrhage, vomiting

## Special Nursing Considerations and Patient Education

- Store in refrigerator.
- Teach patient to
  - notify physician for chest or leg pain, vaginal bleeding.
- Be aware that
  - medication may increase risk of endometrial carcinoma, gallbladder disease, MI, pulmonary embolism, thrombophlebitis.

# Ethacrynic Acid

**Brand Name**
Edecrin

**Actions**
Diuretic; hinders chloride and sodium reabsorption.
Onset evident: PO 30 minutes; IV 5 minutes

**Uses**
Acute pulmonary edema; ascites caused by
cirrhosis; edema associated with congestive heart
failure, renal disease; lymphedema, malignancy

**Contraindications**
Anuria, azotemia, cirrhosis, electrolyte depletion,
hepatic coma, infants, jaundice, oliguria, renal
dysfunction, watery diarrhea. *Use with caution:*
Diabetes, gout, hepatic dysfunction

**Interactions**
Alcohol, aminoglycosides, antihypertensives,
digitalis, lithium, narcotics, salicylates,
vancomycin, warfarin

**Dose**
*Adult*  PO: Initial dose: 50–100 mg; *maintenance*
dose: 50–100 mg qd-bid
*Peds*  PO: Initial dose: 25 mg; increase by 25 mg
increments to individualized maintenance
dose

**Forms**
Sodium injection, tablets

## Adverse Effects

Agranulocytosis, anorexia, diarrhea, dysphagia, headache, hyperuricemia, hypokalemia, hyponatremia, jaundice, metabolic alkalosis, nausea, vomiting, weakness

## Special Nursing Considerations and Patient Education

- Do not administer IM or SC.
- Monitor blood pressure (until dosage is stabilized), diuresis, hematuria, I&O, tarry stools.
- Teach patient
  - to take after meals or with food to decrease GI upset.
  - regarding diuretic effect.
  - to include potassium-rich foods in diet (see Appendix F).
  - to notify physician for signs of electrolyte imbalance (e.g., anorexia, confusion, drowsiness, headache, nausea, thirst, vomiting).

# Ethchlorvynol

**Brand Name**
Placidyl

**Actions**
Anticonvulsant, CNS depressant, hypnotic, muscle relaxant. Onset evident in 30 minutes.

**Uses**
Anxiety, insomnia, tension, to achieve sedation

**Contraindications**
*Meds* Alcohol, CNS depressants
*Other* Children, history of porphyria. *Use with caution:* Hepatic or renal dysfunction, uncontrolled pain

**Interactions**
Antihistamines, hypnotics, MAO inhibitors, narcotics, oral anticoagulants, sedatives, tricyclic antidepressants, tranquilizers

**Dose**
*Adult* 100 mg–1 gm hs

**Forms**
Capsules

**Adverse Effects**
Blurred vision, dizziness, facial numbness, headache, hives, hypotension, nausea, urticaria, vomiting

**Special Nursing Considerations
and Patient Education**
- Store medication in light-resistant container.
- If used as a hypnotic, administer 15–30 minutes prior to bedtime.
- Discontinue for hemorrhage, rash.
- Use caution when administering to a patient with suicidal potential; ensure patient swallows dose.
- Be aware that
  - medication may be habit-forming; when discontinued, decrease dosage gradually.
  - tolerance can develop.
- Teach patient
  - that medication may cause aftertaste, pale stools, dark urine.
  - to be cautious when driving or involved in potentially hazardous tasks.

# Ethosuximide

**Brand Name**
Zarontin

**Actions**
Anticonvulsant, antiepileptic; depresses motor cortex and elevates CNS threshold to convulsive stimuli

**Uses**
Petit mal seizures

**Contraindications**
Chloramphenicol, medications that depress bone-marrow function. *Use with caution:* Blood dyscrasias, epilepsy, hepatic or renal dysfunction, psychologic abnormalities

**Interactions**
Amphetamines, anticonvulsants, antipsychotics, tricyclic antidepressants

**Dose**
*Adult* Individualized; 250 mg bid
*Peds* 3–6 yr: 250 mg/day in divided doses
over 6 yr: Same as adult

**Forms**
Capsules, syrup

**Adverse Effects**
Anorexia, ataxia, depression, diarrhea, dizziness, drowsiness, euphoria, headache, hematuria, irritability, lupus erythematosus, mood changes, nausea, Stevens-Johnson syndrome, thrombocytopenia, urinary frequency, vomiting, weight loss

## Special Nursing Considerations
## and Patient Education

- When discontinued, decrease dosage gradually.
- Maintain serum level of medication at 40–80 µg/cc to control seizures.
- Advise family regarding possibility of aggressiveness, hypochondriacal behavior, or transient personality changes.
- Teach patient
  - to be cautious when driving or involved in potentially hazardous tasks.
  - to take with food or milk to decrease gastric irritation.
  - to carry some type of Medic Alert card or bracelet.
  - notify physician for rash.

# Ethoxazolamide

**Brand Name**

Cardrase, Ethamide

**Actions**

Diuretic, carbonic anhydrase inhibitor. Onset evident in 2 hours.

**Uses**

Adjunct treatment of convulsions, edema, glaucoma; decreases intraocular pressure pre-op

**Contraindications**

Addison's disease, allergy to sulfonamides, chronic pulmonary disease, hepatic or renal dysfunction, hyperchloremic acidosis, hypokalemia, hyponatremia. *Use with caution:* Chronic, noncongestive, closed-angle glaucoma; diabetes; gout; hypercalciuria

**Interactions**

Amphetamines, corticosteroids, digitalis glycosides, insulin, lithium, oral hypoglycemics, phenobarbital, phenytoin, procainamide, quinidine, salicylates, tricyclic antidepressants

**Dose**

*Adult* Edema: 62.5–125 mg/day qod 3 days/week; glaucoma: 62.5–250 mg bid–qid

**Forms**

Tablets

**Adverse Effects**

Acidosis, anorexia, constipation, diarrhea, disorientation, dizziness, drowsiness, fatigue, hypokalemia, nausea, paresthesia, polyuria, thirst, vomiting, weight loss

## Special Nursing Considerations and Patient Education
- Monitor I&O, weight.
- Teach patient
  - to be cautious when driving or involved in potentially hazardous tasks.

# Fluocinonide

**Brand Name**
Lidex, Lidex-E, Topsyn

**Actions**
Anti-inflammatory, antipruritic, corticosteroid, vasoconstrictor

**Uses**
Dermatoses

**Contraindications**
Fungal infections, markedly impaired circulation, vaccinia, varicella

**Interactions**
None

**Dose**
*Adult* Apply to areas tid-qid

**Forms**
Cream, gel, ointment

**Adverse Effects**
Acne, electrolyte/fluid disturbances, hypertension, hypopigmentation, nausea

**Special Nursing Considerations
and Patient Education**
- Do not use occlusive dressings on infected
  lesions.
- Be aware that
  - this medication may be absorbed systemically if
    applied to a large body area for prolonged
    periods.
- Teach patient
  - to avoid getting medication in eyes.

# Fluphenazine

**Brand Name**
Prolixin, Permitil

**Actions**
Antiemetic, antipsychotic, major tranquilizer.
Onset evident: PO 1 week; parenteral 24–72 hours.

**Uses**
Acute or chronic schizophrenia; involutional,
senile, or toxic psychosis; psychomotor agitation

**Contraindications**
*Meds* Alcohol, CNS depressants
*Other* Bone-marrow disorders, brain damage,
children under 12, hepatic or renal
dysfunction. *Use with caution:* Asthma,
emphysema, epilepsy, peptic ulcer

**Interactions**
Amphetamines, antacids, anticoagulants,
antidepressants, antihistamines, guanethidine,
hypnotics, narcotics, quinidine, sedatives,
tranquilizers

**Dose**
*Adult* PO: Hydrochloride: 2.5–20 mg/day; decanoate,
enanthate: 25 mg IM/SC; *maintenance* dose
individualized: q 2 weeks
*Peds* Children over 12: Same as adult

**Forms**
Decanoate injection; enanthate injection;
hydrochloride concentrate, elixir, injection, and
tablets; repeat-action tablets

## Adverse Effects

Blurred vision, dizziness, drowsiness, dry mouth, extrapyramidal symptoms, headache, hypotension, nausea

## Special Nursing Considerations and Patient Education

- Protect medication from light.
- Discard unused medication if its color is darker than light amber.
- Use dry needle and syringe for injection (decanoate/enanthate utilize sesame seed oil as a vehicle).
- Have patient remain recumbent for ½ hour after injection.
- Dilute oral concentrate.
- Offer hard candy (regular or sugar-free) to relieve dry mouth.
- When discontinued, decrease dosage gradually.
- Monitor blood pressure, renal function with long-term administration.
- Teach patient
  - that medication may turn urine brown, pink, or red.
  - to be cautious when driving or involved in potentially hazardous tasks.
  - to notify physician for hemorrhage, jaundice, rash, sore throat, tremors, vision impairment, weakness.

# Flurandrenolide

**Brand Name**
Cordran

**Actions**
Anti-inflammatory, antipruritic, vasoconstrictor

**Uses**
Dermatoses

**Contraindications**
Impaired circulation, ophthalmic use, vaccinia, varicella

**Interactions**
None

**Dose**
*Adult* Apply bid-tid
*Peds* Same as adult

**Forms**
Cream, lotion, ointment, tape

**Adverse Effects**
Dry skin, hypertrichosis, miliaria, pruritus, skin maceration

## Special Nursing Considerations and Patient Education

- Always cleanse area before applying to avoid accumulation of medication.
- Teach patient
  - to continue medication for several days following resolution of lesions to ensure healing.

# Flurazepam HCl

**Brand Name**
Dalmane

**Actions**
Hypnotic. Onset evident in 30–60 minutes.

**Uses**
Insomnia

**Contraindications**
*Meds* Alcohol
*Other* Children under 15, depression, hepatic or renal
dysfunction. *Use with caution:* Allergy to
chemically related medications, epilepsy,
pulmonary disease

**Interactions**
Anticonvulsants, antidepressants, CNS
depressants, hypnotics, MAO inhibitors, narcotics,
sedatives, tranquilizers, tricyclic antidepressants

**Dose**
*Adult* 15–30 mg hs
*Peds* Over 15 years: Same as adult

**Forms**
Capsules

**Adverse Effects**
Ataxia, diarrhea, dizziness, headache, light-
headedness, nausea, sedation, vomiting

## Special Nursing Considerations
## and Patient Education
- Protect medication from heat and direct light.
- Be aware that
  - effects may be cumulative.
  - dependence is possible; when discontinued, decrease dosage gradually.
- Teach patient
  - to decrease use of caffeine and cigarettes/cigars because of their stimulating effect.
  - to be cautious when driving or involved in potentially hazardous tasks.

# Furosemide

## Brand Name
Lasix

## Actions
Diuretic; hinders chloride and sodium reabsorption.
Onset evident: PO 20–60 minutes; IV 5 minutes.

## Uses
Ascites, cirrhosis, congestive heart failure,
nephrosis, pulmonary edema, renal dysfunction

## Contraindications
Anuria, electrolyte depletion, jaundice (children,
infants), oliguria, renal dysfunction. *Use with
caution:* Allergy to sulfonamides, diabetes, gout,
hearing impairment, hepatic dysfunction,
hyperuricemia, lupus erythematosus, pancreatitis

## Interactions
Alcohol, amikacin, capreomycin, chloroquine,
ethacrynic acid, kanamycin, lithium, neomycin,
ototoxic drugs, oxyphenbutazone, phenylbutazone,
streptomycin, vancomycin, viomycin

## Dose
*Adult*  PO: 20–80 mg as single dose in morning
(dosage may be carefully titrated up to 600
mg/day); IM, IV: 20–40 mg as single dose in
morning
*Peds*  PO: 2 mg/kg/day; IM, IV: 1 mg/kg/day;
*maximum* dose: 6 mg/kg/day

## Forms
Injection, liquid, tablets

## Adverse Effects

Blurred vision, diarrhea, hyperuricemia, hypokalemia, hyponatremia, muscle cramps, nausea, paresthesia, orthostatic hypotension, transient deafness, vomiting

## Special Nursing Considerations and Patient Education

- Protect medication from direct light.
- Administer IV dose slowly over 1–2 minutes.
- Inject IM dose slowly into deep muscles.
- Observe for hypersensitivity to sulfonamides (patients may experience cross-allergenicity).
- Monitor blood pressure; blood levels of carbon dioxide, electrolytes, serum BUN; I&O; vital signs; weight.
- Discontinue for hearing impairment, hypokalemia, hyponatremia.
- Be aware that
  - patient may need potassium supplements or changes in salt intake.
- Teach patient
  - that medication may cause sweet taste in mouth.
  - to change position slowly to decrease postural hypotension.
  - to be cautious during hot weather or strenuous exercise to decrease possibility of orthostatic hypotension.

# Glutethimide

**Brand Name**
Doriden

**Actions**
CNS depressant, hypnotic, sedative. Onset evident in 15–30 minutes.

**Uses**
Insomnia

**Contraindications**
*Meds* Alcohol, CNS depressants
*Other* Children, emotional disorders, glaucoma, porphyria. *Use with caution:* Cardiac dysrhythmias, pain, prostatic hypertrophy, pyloroduodenal obstruction, renal dysfunction

**Interactions**
Analgesics, anticholinergics, antidepressants, antihistamines, hypnotics, narcotics, oral anticoagulants, sedatives, tranquilizers

**Dose**
*Adult* 250–500 mg hs

**Forms**
Capsules, tablets

**Adverse Effects**
Blood dycrasias, blurred vision, dizziness, headache, hiccoughs, light-headedness, nausea, paradoxical excitation, rash

**Special Nursing Considerations
and Patient Education**
- Discontinue for rash.
- Be aware that
  - effectiveness of medication can be decreased if
    patient is in pain.
  - dependence is possible; when discontinued,
    decrease dosage gradually.
- Teach patient
  - to be cautious when driving or involved in
    potentially hazardous tasks.

# Griseofulvin

**Brand Name**
Fulvicin, Grisactin

**Actions**
Antibiotic, fungistatic; hinders metabolic activities of fungus

**Uses**
Athlete's foot, ringworm

**Contraindications**
Candidiasis, hepatic or hepatocellular failure, porphyria, systemic mycoses. *Use with caution:* Allergy to penicillin, depression, lupus erythematosus

**Interactions**
Alcohol, barbiturates, oral anticoagulants

**Dose**
*Adult* Ultramicrosize: 250–500 mg/day; microsize: 500 mg–1 gm/day
*Peds* Ultramicrosize: 5 mg/kg/day; microsize: 10 mg/kg/day

**Forms**
Microsize: capsules or tablets, suspension; ultramicrosize: tablets

**Adverse Effects**
Confusion, diarrhea, dry mouth, fatigue, GI distress, headache, insomnia, leukopenia, paresthesia, proteinuria, urticaria

## Special Nursing Considerations
## and Patient Education
- Teach patient
  - to maintain good personal hygiene.
  - that medication may cause photosensitivity.
  - to ingest a diet high in fat to enhance
    absorption.
  - that treatment must be continued for 2 weeks to
    6 months after symptoms are gone.
  - to notify physician for fever, malaise, sore
    throat.
  - to take medication after meals to decrease GI
    distress.

# Guaifenesin

**Brand Name**
    Robitussin

**Actions**
    Expectorant; lessens adhesiveness and viscosity
    of respiratory secretions

**Uses**
    Cough relief, respiratory congestion

**Contraindications**
    Hypersensitivity

**Interactions**
    None

**Dose**
Adult   100–200 mg q3–4h
*Peds*   2–6 yr: 25–50 mg q3–4h
        6–12 yr: 50–100 mg q3–4h

**Forms**
    Capsules, syrup, tablets

**Adverse Effects**
    Drowsiness, nausea, vomiting

## Special Nursing Considerations
## and Patient Education
- Maintain patient's level of hydration.
- Teach patient
  - to decrease smoking and talking to soothe
    irritated throat.

# Guaifenesin/Theophylline

**Brand Name**
Quibron

**Actions**
Bronchodilator, expectorant, sympathomimetic.
Onset evident in 1 hour.

**Uses**
Asthmatic bronchospasm, chronic bronchitis,
emphysema

**Contraindications**
Hypersensitivity. *Use with caution:* Acute cardiac
disease, cor pulmonale, glaucoma, gout, hepatic or
renal disease, hypertension, hyperthyroidism,
hypoxemia, myocardial damage, neonates,
porphyria, prostatic hypertrophy

**Interactions**
Allopurinol, anticoagulants, chlordiazepoxide,
cimetidine, clindamycin, digitalis, erythromycin,
furosemide, lincomycin, lithium, phenobarbital,
phenytoin, propranolol, sympathomimetics

**Dose**
*Adult* 150 mg q6-8h or 15-30 cc q6h
*Peds* Under 9 yr: 4-6 mg of theophylline/kg q6-8h;
9-12 yr: 4-5 mg of theophylline/kg q6-8h

**Forms**
Capsules, liquid

**Adverse Effects**
CNS stimulation, dizziness, gastric upset,
headache, insomnia, nausea, tachycardia, vomiting

**Special Nursing Considerations
and Patient Education**
- Monitor I&O, vital signs.
- Administer after meals and with a glass of water to decrease GI irritation.
- Teach patient to
  - be cautious when driving or involved in potentially hazardous tasks.
  - not take nonprescription medications without conferring with physician.
  - decrease intake of caffeine.

# Guanethidine Sulfate

**Brand Name**
Ismelin

**Actions**
Antihypertensive, postganglionic adrenergic-blocking agent; decreases blood vessel constriction. Onset evident in 48–72 hours.

**Uses**
Hypertension

**Contraindications**
*Meds*  Alcohol, CNS depressants, MAO inhibitors
*Other*  Congestive heart failure (not originating from hypertension), mild uncomplicated hypertension, pheochromocytoma. *Use with caution:* Cerebrovascular disease; encephalopathy; history of asthma, coronary artery disease, CVA, diarrhea, dyspepsia; nitrogen retention; peptic ulcer; recent MI; renal disease; sinus bradycardia

**Interactions**
Amphetamines, digitalis, oral contraceptives, phenothiazines, propranolol, reserpine, tricyclic antidepressants, vasopressors

**Dose**
*Adult*  10 mg/day; 25–50 mg/day if hospitalized
*Peds*  0.2 mg/kg/day

**Forms**
Tablets

## Adverse Effects

Bradycardia, diarrhea, dizziness, drowsiness, edema, fatigue, impotence, orthostatic hypotension, syncope, weakness, weight gain

## Special Nursing Considerations and Patient Education

- Monitor blood pressure (lying and standing), I&O, neurologic status, weight.
- Adjust salt intake if necessary.
- Be aware that
  - medication is cumulative.
  - this drug may affect dosages of antidiabetic medications.
- Teach patient
  - to notify physician of temperature elevations.
  - to decrease smoking and caffeine intake.
  - to be cautious when driving or involved in potentially hazardous tasks.
  - to change position slowly to decrease orthostatic hypotension.
  - that hot weather or strenuous activities may increase the possibility of orthostatic hypotension.
  - to avoid carbonated beverages or to drink them sparingly.

# Haloperidol

**Brand Name**
   Haldol

**Actions**
   Antipsychotic; inhibits brainstem activity. Onset
   evident: PO 3 weeks; IM 30–45 minutes.

**Uses**
   Acute or chronic psychotic disorders, behavioral
   problems, Gilles de la Tourette's syndrome

**Contraindications**
*Meds* Alcohol, CNS depressants, lithium
*Other* Children under 3 years, comatose patients,
   depression, parkinsonism. *Use with caution:*
   Cardiovascular, hepatic or respiratory
   dysfunction; diabetes; epilepsy; glaucoma

**Interactions**
   Anticonvulsants, antihistamines, barbiturates,
   guanethidine, hypnotics, narcotics, oral
   anticoagulants, sedatives, tranquilizers, tricyclic
   antidepressants

**Dose**
*Adult* PO: 0.5–5 mg bid-tid; IM: 2–5 mg q1–8h;
   individualized doses up to 100 mg may be
   necessary.
*Peds* Over 3 yr: 0.05–0.15 mg/kg/day PO

**Forms**
   Concentrate, injection, tablets

**Adverse Effects**
   Blurred vision, constipation, drowsiness, dry
   mouth, extrapyramidal symptoms, headache,

insomnia, nausea, orthostatic hypotension, tachycardia, vomiting

**Special Nursing Considerations and Patient Education**
- Protect medication from direct light.
- Monitor for fine vermicular tongue movements (may indicate early tardive dyskinesia).
- Dilute concentrate in fluids other than coffee or tea.
- Give injections in upper, outer quadrant of buttocks.
- Have patient lie down for 1 hour after parenteral administration.
- Monitor blood pressure.
- Discontinue for jaundice, tremors, impairment or weakness of vision.
- Be aware that
  - medication is eliminated slowly.
  - medication decreases seizure threshold.
- Teach patient
  - to be cautious when driving or involved in potentially hazardous tasks.
  - to use caution when in the sun because of the possibility of photosensitivity.

# Heparin Sodium Injection

**Brand Name**
Hep-Lock, Lipo-Hepin

**Actions**
Anticoagulant; hinders prothrombin from forming thrombin

**Uses**
Arterial occlusion; atrial fibrillation with embolism; cardiac/vascular surgery; hyperlipemia; pulmonary embolism; thrombophlebitis; adjunct treatment of coronary occlusion with acute MI

**Contraindications**
*Meds* Anesthetics (lumbar block, regional)
*Other* Acute hemorrhage; blood dycrasias; chronic ulcerative colitis; following brain, eye, or spinal cord surgery; hepatic or renal dysfunction; hypertension; peptic ulcer; shock; subacute bacterial endocarditis; suspected intracranial hemorrhage; threatened abortion; tube drainage of small intestine and stomach; visceral carcinoma. *Use with caution:* Alcoholism, allergies, arteriosclerosis, asthma, indwelling catheter, jaundice, menstruation, open wounds, purpura, skin denudation, thrombocytopenia, thrombophlebitis, ulcerative lesions

**Interactions**
ACTH, antihistamines, aspirin, corticosteroids, dextran, diazepam, digitalis, dipyridamole, hydroxychloroquine, ibuprofen, indomethacin, insulin, tetracycline

## Dose
*Adult* IV infusion: 10,000–40,000 U/day; SC–deep: initially, 10,000–20,000 U, then 8,000–10,000 U q8h

*Peds* IV infusion: 50 U/kg; followed by 100 U/kg or 3,333 U/m² 6x/day

## Forms
Injection, pre-filled syringes

## Adverse Effects
Alopecia, chills, ecchymosis, epistaxis, fever, hemarthrosis, hematuria, hemorrhage

## Special Nursing Considerations and Patient Education
- Use trial dose to test for allergic response.
- Verify clotting time, PTT, or APTT prior to administration (dosage is adjusted according to these lab values).
- Avoid IM route since there is a tendency for patient to form hematomas.
- Administer SC via Z-track technique. Do not rub skin before or after SC injection as this may damage tissue. Do not pinch skin or withdraw plunger before administration.
- Monitor clotting time, vital signs; check injection site, stools, and urine for bleeding.
- Be aware that
  - patient is in increased danger of hemorrhage.
- Teach patient to
  - not smoke.
  - carry some type of Medic Alert bracelet or card containing dosage and resource telephone numbers.
  - notify physician of any signs of hemorrhage.

# Hydralazine HCl

**Brand Name**
Apresoline

**Actions**
Antihypertensive; relaxes vascular smooth muscle

**Uses**
Hypertensive conditions

**Contraindications**
Advanced renal disease, angina pectoris, chronic glomerulonephritis, coronary heart disease, rheumatic heart disease with mitral valve involvement. *Use with caution:* Advanced renal damage, coronary artery disease, existing or incipient CVA, lupus erythematosus

**Interactions**
Alcohol, amphetamines, antihypertensives, MAO inhibitors, sympathomimetics

**Dose**
*Adult*  PO: 10 mg qid; gradually increase to 50 mg qid
*Peds*  PO: 0.75 mg/kg/day in 4 divided doses

**Forms**
Injection, tablets

**Adverse Effects**
Anorexia, chest pain, diaphoresis, diarrhea, dizziness, headache, nausea, palpitations, orthostatic hypotension, rheumatoid syndrome, tachycardia, vomiting

## Special Nursing Considerations and Patient Education

- Monitor blood pressure, I&O, mental and neurologic status, renal function, weight.
- Teach patient
  - to be cautious when driving or involved in potentially hazardous tasks.
  - to use caution during cold weather or strenuous exercise because of the possibility of orthostatic hypotension.
  - to notify physician for fever and/or chest or joint pain.

# Hydrochlorothiazide

**Brand Name**
Esidrix, HydroDIURIL, Oretic

**Actions**
Antihypertensive, diuretic; hinders sodium
reabsorption. Onset evident in 2 hours.

**Uses**
Edema, hypertension

**Contraindications**
*Meds* Lithium
*Other* Hypersensitivity to sulfonamide-derived
medications, renal decompensation. *Use with
caution:* Allergy to sulfonamides, diabetes,
gout, hepatic or renal dysfunction,
hypercalcemia, hyperuricemia, lupus
erythematosus, pancreatitis, sympathectomy

**Interactions**
ACTH, antigout drugs, antihypertensives,
corticosteroids, digitalis, insulin, lithium, oral
antidiabetics

**Dose**
*Adult* Edema: 25–200 mg qd; hypertension: 75
mg/day, to be adjusted
*Peds* Under 6 months: 3.3 mg/kg/day in 2 doses; over
6 months: 2.2 mg/kg/day

**Forms**
Tablets

**Adverse Effects**
Anorexia, constipation, diarrhea, dizziness,
headache, hypokalemia, hypotension, nausea,
orthostatic hypotension, paresthesia, vomiting

**Special Nursing Considerations
and Patient Education**
- Monitor blood pressure, electrolytes (particularly serum potassium level), weight.
- Discontinue for electrolyte imbalances.
- Teach patient
  - that medication may cause photosensitivity.
  - to ingest potassium-rich foods (see Appendix F).
  - to be cautious when driving or involved in potentially hazardous tasks.
  - to use caution during hot weather or strenuous exercise because of the possibility of orthostatic hypotension.

# Hydrochlorothiazide/ Spironolactone

**Brand Name**
Aldactazide

**Actions**
Antihypertensive, diuretic; decreases exchangeable sodium

**Uses**
Edema, hypertension

**Contraindications**
Allergies to sulfonamide-derived medications or thiazide diuretics, anuria, hepatic failure, hyperkalemia, renal impairment. *Use with caution:* Diabetes

**Interactions**
ACTH, digitalis, diuretics, glucocorticoids, lithium, potassium supplements

**Dose**
*Adult* Individualized; *average* dose: 1 tablet qid
*Peds* Individualized; *average* dose: 1.65–3.3 mg spironolactone/kg/day

**Forms**
Tablets

**Adverse Effects**
Confusion, diarrhea, dizziness, drowsiness, dry mouth, headache, hyperkalemia, hyponatremia, hypotension, nausea, restlessness, tachycardia, thirst, vertigo, vomiting, weakness

**Special Nursing Considerations
and Patient Education**
- Monitor electrolyte and fluid balance, weight.
- Administer early in morning, after meal, to decrease GI upset.
- Offer hard candy (regular or sugar-free) to relieve dry mouth.
- Teach patient
  - to change position slowly to decrease hypotension.
  - that medication may cause photosensitivity.
  - caution regarding driving or involvement in potentially hazardous tasks.
  - to not take nonprescription medications without conferring with physician.

# Hydroflumethiazide/Reserpine

**Brand Name**
Salutensin

**Actions**
Antihypertensive, diuretic; hinders reabsorption of sodium and chloride in tubules

**Uses**
Hypertension

**Contraindications**
Active peptic ulcer, anuria, children, depression, ECT, oliguria, ulcerative colitis. *Use with caution:* Asthma, diabetes, digitalized patients, gallstones, GI disorders, gout, hyperuricemia, lupus erythematosus, renal insufficiency

**Interactions**
ACTH, anticonvulsants, antihistamines, digitalis, hypnotics, insulin, MAO inhibitors, narcotics, oral anticoagulants, phenothiazines, propranolol, quinidine, sedatives, steroids, tranquilizers

**Dose**
*Adult* Individualized; *average* dose: 1–2 tablets qd–bid

**Forms**
Demi-tablets, tablets

**Adverse Effects**
Anorexia, constipation, depression, diarrhea, dizziness, drowsiness, dry mouth, dyspnea, electrolyte and fluid imbalance, hypokalemia, hypotension, lethargy, nasal congestion, nausea, restlessness, syncope, tachycardia, thirst, vertigo, vomiting

**Special Nursing Considerations
and Patient Education**
- Protect medication from direct light.
- Monitor blood pressure, I&O, pulse, weight.
- Offer hard candy (regular or sugar-free) to relieve dry mouth.
- Administer with meals or milk to decrease GI upset.
- Consult with physician regarding diet.
- Be aware that
  - generally, this drug is not used for initial therapy.
- Teach patient
  - that medication may cause photosensitivity.
  - to be cautious when driving or involved in potentially hazardous tasks.
  - to change position slowly to decrease hypotension.
  - to not take nonprescription medications without conferring with physician.

# Hydroxyzine HCl, Hydroxyzine Pamoate

**Brand Name**
  Atarax, Vistaril

**Actions**
  Anticholinergic, antiemetic, antihistamine,
  sedative, tranquilizer; depresses brainstem
  (reticular formation) and hypothalamus. Onset
  evident in 15–30 minutes.

**Uses**
  Allergic dermatoses, anxiety, nausea, psychomotor
  agitation, tension, urticaria

**Contraindications**
  Alcohol, CNS depressants. *Use with caution:*
  Epilepsy

**Interactions**
  Analgesics, anticholinesterase drugs,
  anticoagulants, antihistamines, barbiturates,
  hypnotics, narcotics, phenothiazines, sedatives

**Dose**
*Adult*  PO: 25–100 mg tid-qid
*Peds*  Under 6 yr: 50 mg/day PO in divided doses
    Over 6 yr: 50–100 mg/day PO in divided doses

**Forms**
  Hydroxyzine hydrochloride capsules, injections,
  syrup, and tablets; hydroxyzine pamoate capsules,
  injection, and suspension

**Adverse Effects**
  Drowsiness, dry mouth, headache, tremors

## Special Nursing Considerations and Patient Education

- Protect medication from light.
- Shake suspension well prior to administering.
- Administer IM injections slowly into deep muscles (buttocks for adults, midlateral thigh for children) to prevent nerve injury.
- Be aware that
  - tolerance can develop.
- Teach patient to
  - be cautious when driving or involved in potentially hazardous tasks.
  - decrease caffeine intake because of its stimulant effect.

# Ibuprofen

**Brand Name**
Motrin, Advil

**Actions**
Analgesic, anti-inflammatory, antipyretic. Onset evident in 1 hour.

**Uses**
Menstrual pain, osteoarthritis, rheumatoid arthritis

**Contraindications**
Allergy to aspirin, angiodermatitis, aspirin-induced bronchospasm, children under 14, nasal polyps. *Use with caution:* Cardiovascular decompensation, coagulation disorders, congestive heart failure, peptic ulcer, renal dysfunction, upper GI tract disorders.

**Interactions**
Alcohol, anticoagulants, aspirin, phenobarbital, phenytoin, sulfonamides, sulfonylureas

**Dose**
*Adult* 300–400 mg tid–qid; *maximum* dose: 2,400 mg/day

**Forms**
Tablets

**Adverse Effects**
Blurred vision, constipation, cramps, diarrhea, dizziness, dyspepsia, headache, pruritus, tinnitus

**Special Nursing Considerations
and Patient Education**
- Administer medication with food to decrease GI distress.
- Teach patient
  - to be cautious when driving or involved in potentially hazardous tasks.
  - notify physician for blurred vision, edema, skin rash, tarry stools, weight gain.

# Imipramine HCl

**Brand Name**
  Tofranil

**Actions**
  Antidepressant, antipsychotic; hinders re-uptake of
  norepinephrine

**Uses**
  Endogenous or manic depression, involutional
  psychoses

**Contraindications**
*Meds*  Alcohol, MAO inhibitors
*Other*  Narrow-angle glaucoma, recent MI. *Use with
  caution:* Alcoholism, asthma, cardiovascular or
  hepatic dysfunction, diabetes, epilepsy,
  glaucoma, hyperthyroidism, intraocular
  pressure increase, prostatic hypertrophy,
  urinary retention

**Interactions**
  Amphetamines, anticholinergics, anticonvulsants.
  antihistamines, antihypertensives, barbiturates,
  clonidine, CNS depressants, estrogens,
  ethchlorvynol, guanethidine, hypnotics, levodopa,
  narcotics, quinidine, sedatives, sympathomimetics,
  thyroid preparations, tranquilizers

**Dose**
*Adult*  PO: 50 mg bid; increase to *maximum* of 200
  mg/day
*Peds*  PO: 25 mg/day 1 hr before hs

**Forms**
  Injection, tablets

## Adverse Effects

Anorexia, blurred vision, bone-marrow depression, disorientation, dizziness, drowsiness, dry mouth, dysrhythmias, hallucinations, headache, nausea, paresthesia, seizures, tachycardia, urinary retention, vomiting

## Special Nursing Considerations
## and Patient Education

- Protect medication from light.
- Monitor I&O, vital signs, weight.
- Use caution when administering to a patient with suicidal potential; ensure patient swallows dose.
- Offer hard candy (regular or sugar-free) to relieve dry mouth.
- Be aware that
  - tolerance can develop; when discontinued, decrease dosage gradually.
- Teach patient
  - to change position slowly to decrease hypotension.
  - to be cautious when driving or involved in potentially hazardous tasks.
  - that medication may cause a peculiar taste in mouth or photosensitivity.
  - to not take any nonprescription drugs without notifying physician.

# Indomethacin

**Brand Name**
Indocin

**Actions**
Analgesic, anti-inflammatory, antipyretic; blocks prostaglandin biosynthesis. Onset evident in 4–24 hours.

**Uses**
Degenerative joint disease of the hip, gout, gouty or rheumatoid arthritis, rheumatoid spondylitis

**Contraindications**
Active gastritis, children, enteritis, ileitis, nasal polyps associated with aspirin hypersensitivity, peptic ulcer, ulcerative colitis. *Use with caution:* Epilepsy, GI disorders, hemophilia, mental illness, parkinsonism, renal disease

**Interactions**
Aspirin, corticosteroids, furosemide, oral anticoagulants, phenylbutazone, probenicid, salicylates, sulfonamides, thyroid preparations

**Dose**
*Adult* 25 mg bid-tid

**Forms**
Capsules

**Adverse Effects**
Blurred vision, diarrhea, dizziness, drowsiness, headache, nausea, vomiting

## Special Nursing Considerations and Patient Education

- Protect medication from direct light.
- Teach patient
  - to be cautious when driving or involved in potentially hazardous tasks.
  - to take with antacids, food, or after meals to decrease stomach irritation.
  - that this is a toxic medication and to take exactly as directed.
  - to notify physician for blurred vision or tarry stools.

# Insulin

**Brand Name**
Iletin (Regular), Iletin II (Regular), Insulin (Regular)

**Actions**
Antidiabetic, antihyperglycemic; necessary for amino acid and monosaccharide molecule transport. Onset evident in ½-1 hour.

**Uses**
Diabetes, diabetic coma

**Contraindications**
None. *Use with caution:* Fever, hepatic or renal dysfunction, hyper- or hypothyroidism, infections, nausea, vomiting

**Interactions**
Alcohol, anabolic steroids, corticosteroids, epinephrine, guanethidine, MAO inhibitors, oral contraceptives, phenylbutazone, propranolol, sulfinpyrazone, tetracycline, thiazide diuretics, thyroid replacement

**Dose**
*Adult* Individualized; *average* dose: 50–150 U/day
*Peds* Individualized; *average* dose: 1–4 U/kg/day

**Forms**
Injection

**Adverse Effects**
Anxiety, diaphoresis, hypersensitivity or resistance to insulin, hypoglycemia, lassitude, nausea, tremulousness, visual disturbances

## Special Nursing Considerations
## and Patient Education

- Protect medication from heat and light.
- Check expiration date on label.
- Follow administration directions precisely.
- Verify that syringe gradations are appropriate to strength of insulin preparation.
- Administer injections SC into loose connective tissue.
- Refrigerate stock supply.
- Recognize the difference between this type and other types of insulin.
- Be aware that
  - insulin vial currently in use is stable at room temperature up to 1 month.
  - medication should be clear as water.
  - 1 unit of insulin will promote metabolism of approximately 1.5 gm of dextrose.
- Mix with other insulins as follows:
  - Lente Insulin (1:1): mix immediately prior to administration
  - NPH Insulin (any ratio): mix immediately prior to administration
  - Protamine Zinc (any ratio): prepare mixture immediately prior to injection.

*(continued)*

# Insulin (continued)

- Teach patient
  - to maintain prescribed fluid intake and diet.
  - to carry sugar at all times.
  - to self-test urine.
  - to self-administer medication; ask for return demonstration.
  - that medication must be taken as directed and carried on person when traveling.
  - to use caution during strenuous exercise; dosage adjustment may be required.
  - to maintain good personal hygiene to prevent infections
  - to notify physician of illness.
  - to not take any new medications without contacting physician.
  - to carry some type of Medic Alert card or bracelet.

# NOTES

# Isocarboxazid

**Brand Name**
  Marplan

**Actions**
  Antidepressant, MAO inhibitor. Onset evident in
  1–4 weeks.

**Uses**
  Endogenous or reactive depression

**Contraindications**
*Meds*  Alcohol, CNS depressants, general anesthesia,
  narcotics, sympathomimetics, tricyclic
  antidepressants
*Other*  Arteriosclerosis, atonic colitis, cardiovascular
  or renal dysfunction, cerebrovascular disease,
  children under 16, congestive heart failure,
  epilepsy, history of hepatic disease,
  hypernatremia, hypertension, hyperthyroid,
  paranoid schizophrenia, pheochromocytoma.
  *Use with caution:* Angina, diabetes, glaucoma

**Interactions**
  Antihistamines, antihypertensives, appetite
  suppressants, barbiturates, hypoglycemics

**Dose**
*Adult*  30 mg/day

**Forms**
  Tablets

**Adverse Effects**
  Agitation, blurred vision, confusion, constipation,
  dizziness, drowsiness, dry mouth, hypertensive
  crises, orthostatic hypotension, weakness,
  weight gain

**Special Nursing Considerations and Patient Education**

- Observe diabetic patients for signs of hypoglycemia.
- Monitor blood pressure.
- Be aware that
  - there must be a 2 week period without MAO inhibitors before administration of *tricyclic antidepressants*.
- Offer hard candy (regular or sugar-free) to relieve dry mouth.
- Teach patient
  - to eliminate foods high in tryptophan and tyramine from diet because of their toxic effects (see Appendix F).
  - to continue diet restrictions for 2 weeks after medication is discontinued.
  - that medication may cause photosensitivity.
  - notify physician for blurred vision, chest pain, headache, jaundice, nausea, neck stiffening, pupil dilation, vomiting.
  - to be cautious when driving or involved in potentially hazardous tasks.

# Isoproterenol HCl

**Brand Name**
Isuprel, Medihaler-Iso, Norisodrine

**Actions**
Bronchodilator, cardiac stimulant

**Uses**
Adams-Stokes syndrome, asystole or atrioventricular heart block, bronchial asthma, bronchitis, pulmonary emphysema or hypertension, shock, tachycardia, ventricular dysrhythmias from A-V block

**Contraindications**
*Meds* Epinephrine, MAO inhibitors, tricyclic antidepressants
*Other* Cardiac dysrhythmias with tachycardia, coronary blood flow insufficiency or sclerosis, history of tachycardia, hyperexcitability, hypertension. *Use with caution:* Cardiac disease, diabetes, heart block, hypertension, hyperthyroidism, tuberculosis, valvular stenosis

**Interactions**
Digitalis, ephedrine, propranolol, sympathomimetics

**Dose**
*Adult* Inhalation: 1–2 inhalations 4–6x/day
Sublingual: 10–20 mg tid–qid; IV: 0.01–0.02 mg prn
*Peds* Individualized: 5–10 mg tid–qid

**Forms**
Inhalation powder and solution, injection, sublingual tablets

## Adverse Effects

Angina, bronchial edema, diaphoresis, flushing, headache, insomnia, nervousness, palpitations, precordial pain, tachycardia, tremors

## Special Nursing Considerations and Patient Education

- Protect medication from direct light.
- Discard inhalation solution if brownish.
- This medication has precise directions for administration; follow exactly as indicated.
- Correct existing hypovolemia prior to administering this drug.
- Do not administer if precordial angina pectoris is present.
- Monitor blood pressure, pulse.
- Notify physician of palpitations, other cardiac or respiratory problems.
- Be aware that
  - tolerance may develop.
- Teach patient
  - that saliva and sputum may turn pink after inhalation.

# Isosorbide Dinitrate

**Brand Name**
Isordil, Iso-Bid, Sorbide

**Actions**
Coronary vasodilator; relaxes vascular smooth muscle. Onset evident: PO 15–30 minutes; sublingual 2–5 minutes; sustained-release 30 minutes.

**Uses**
Angina pectoris

**Contraindications**
Sensitivity to hypotension. *Use with caution:* Anemia, glaucoma, hyperthyroidism, intracranial pressure, MI

**Interactions**
Alcohol, antihypertensives, sympathomimetics

**Dose**
*Adult* 5–30 mg tid–qid; sustained-release: 40 mg q6–12h

**Forms**
Chewable, sublingual, and sustained-release tablets; sustained-release capsules

**Adverse Effects**
Blurred vision, dizziness, flushing, nausea, orthostatic hypotension, reflex tachycardia, vascular headache, vertigo, vomiting

**Special Nursing Considerations
and Patient Education**
- Protect medication from heat and light.
- Store medication in original containers.
- When discontinued, decrease dosage gradually.
- Be aware that
  - tolerance can develop.
- Teach patient to
  - notify physician if pain is not relieved by 3
    tablets after 30 minutes.
  - change position slowly to decrease hypotension.
  - eliminate smoking when using sublingual
    tablets.
  - not swallow sublingual tablets.
  - avoid stress as much as possible.
  - use caution in cold weather and during
    strenuous exercise because of potential
    orthostatic hypotension.
  - notify physician for blurred vision, rash.

# Isoxsuprine HCl

**Brand Name**
Vasodilan

**Actions**
Cerebral or peripheral vasodilator; inhibits smooth uterine and vascular muscles. Onset evident in 1 hour.

**Uses**
Arteriosclerotic disease, Buerger's disease, cerebrovascular insufficiency, dysmenorrhea, peripheral vascular spasm, Raynaud's disease

**Contraindications**
Arterial hemorrhage, hypotension and tachycardia (parenteral forms), postpartum patients. *Use with caution:* Circulatory impairment of heart or brain, hypotension, tachycardia

**Interactions**
Tricyclic antidepressants

**Dose**
*Adult* PO: 10–20 mg tid–qid; IM: 5–10 mg bid–tid

**Forms**
Injection, tablets

**Adverse Effects**
Dizziness, flushing, light-headedness, nausea, nervousness, palpitations, orthostatic hypotension, rash, vomiting

## Special Nursing Considerations and Patient Education

- Monitor blood pressure, pulse; with threatened abortion, monitor duration, frequency, intensity of contractions.
- Discontinue for rash.
- Teach patient to
  - change position slowly to decrease hypotension.
  - be cautious when driving or involved in potentially hazardous tasks.
  - decrease smoking to enhance effectiveness of medication.

# Levodopa

**Brand Name**

Larodopa, Sinemet

**Actions**

Changes into dopamine in CNS. Onset evident in 2–3 weeks.

**Uses**

Carbon monoxide or manganese poisoning, idiopathic or postencephalitic parkinsonism

**Contraindications**

*Meds* Adrenergics, MAO inhibitors

*Other* Blood dyscrasias, children under 12, history of melanoma, hypertension, narrow-angle glaucoma, suspicious skin lesions. *Use with caution:* Bronchial asthma; cardiovascular disease; convulsions; CVA; diabetes; dysrhythmias; emphysema; endocrine, hepatic, or renal disorders; history of MI; hypertension; neuroses; physiologic disorders with an organic base; psychoses; wide-angle glaucoma

**Interactions**

Amphetamines, anticholinergics, antihypertensives, antimuscarinics, ephedrine, guanethidine, haloperidol, hypoglycemics, MAO inhibitors, methyldopa, phenothiazines, phenylephrine, phenytoin, pyridoxine, reserpine, sympathomimetics, thioxanthenes, tranquilizers, vitamin $B_6$

**Dose**

*Adult* Initial dose: 0.5–1 gm/day in 2 or more doses with food; increase dose every 3–7 days as

tolerated; usual therapeutic dose should not
exceed 8 gm/day
*Peds* Over 12: same as adult

## Forms
Capsules, tablets

## Adverse Effects
Adventitious, choreiform, or dystonic movements;
akinesia; anorexia; anxiety; bruxism; constipation;
depression; diarrhea; dysphagia; fatigue;
grimacing; hypertension; insomnia; orthostatic
hypotension; palpitations; weakness

## Special Nursing Considerations
and Patient Education
- Protect medication from direct light.
- Monitor for behavior changes, indications of
  suicide ideation, vital signs.
- Teach patient
  - to not take vitamins that contain 10–25 mg of
    vitamin B₆.
  - to take with meals to decrease irritation.
  - to be cautious when driving or involved in
    potentially hazardous tasks.
  - to use caution during strenuous exercise if has a
    history of cardiac problems.
  - to change position slowly to decrease
    hypotension.
  - that medication may turn perspiration and/or
    urine pink or red.

# Levothyroxine Sodium

**Brand Name**
Synthroid, Levoid

**Actions**
Thyroid preparation. Onset evident in 1–3 weeks.

**Uses**
Hypothyroidism

**Contraindications**
Cardiac disease, MI, thyrotoxicosis. *Use with caution:* Adrenocortical insufficiency, angina pectoris, arteriosclerosis, cardiovascular dysfunction, diabetes, hypertension, panhypopituitarism

**Interactions**
Cholestyramine, insulin, ketamine hydrochloride, oral anticoagulants or antidiabetics, phenytoin, sympathomimetics, tricyclic antidepressants

**Dose**
*Adult* PO: 0.1 mg/day; increase by 0.05–0.1 mg/day q1–3 weeks
*Peds* PO: 0.05 mg/day; increase by 0.025–0.05 mg/day until desired response is obtained

**Forms**
Injection, tablets

**Adverse Effects**
Constipation, headache, muscle aches, sedation, weight gain

**Special Nursing Considerations
and Patient Education**
- Protect medication from light.
- Give solution immediately after preparing it.
- Do not use bacteriostatic sodium chloride for injections.
- Be aware that
  - medication is usually given as a single dose before breakfast.

# Lidocaine HCl (IV Injection)

**Brand Name**

Xylocaine Hydrochloride

**Actions**

Anesthetic, antidysrhythmic; decreases refractory period. Onset evident in 2 minutes.

**Uses**

Ventricular dysrhythmia

**Contraindications**

Adams-Stokes Syndrome; allergy to amide in local anesthetics; atrioventricular, intraventricular, or sinoatrial heart block; Wolff-Parkinson-White syndrome. *Use with caution:* Congestive heart failure, hepatic or renal dysfunction, hypoxia, respiratory distress, shock

**Interactions**

Phenytoin, procainamide, propranolol

**Dose**

*Adult* Infusion: 20–50 $\mu$g/kg of body weight/minute (1–4 mg/minute)

*Peds* Physician determined; 10–50 $\mu$g/kg of body weight/minute

**Forms**

Injection (with dextrose or epinephrine)

**Adverse Effects**

Blurred vision, bradycardia, disorientation, dizziness, drowsiness, euphoria, involuntary movements, nausea, paresthesia, respiratory difficulty, restlessness, tinnitus, tremors, vomiting

## Special Nursing Considerations and Patient Education
- Do not add to blood transfusion assembly.
- Monitor blood pressure, cardiac depressant effects, EKG, neurotoxic effects.
- Discontinue for prolongation of PR interval and QRS complex or aggravation of dysrhythmia.
- Be aware that
  - a possible cross allergy between procainamide or quinidine exists.
  - effects are cumulative.

# Lithium Carbonate

**Brand Name**
Eskalith, Lithane, Lithobid, Lithonate, Lithotabs

**Actions**
Antimanic; alters neuronal characteristics. Onset evident in 1–3 weeks.

**Uses**
Psychoses (manic-depression)

**Contraindications**
Brain damage, cardiovascular dysfunction, children under 12, renal disease, pregnant women. *Use with caution:* CNS disorders, dehydration, diabetes, hypotension, hypothyroidism, low-sodium diet, renal insufficiency, severe infections, urinary retention

**Interactions**
Acetazolamide, aminophylline, chlorpromazine, diuretics, dyphylline, haloperidol, iodide preparations, mannitol, oxtriphylline, phenytoin, sodium bicarbonate, theophylline

**Dose**
*Adult* Initial dose: 600 mg tid; *maintenance* dose: 300 mg tid–qid
*Peds* Over 12: same as adult

**Forms**
Capsules, sustained-release tablets, tablets

**Adverse Effects**
Diarrhea, dizziness, drowsiness, dry mouth, extrapyramidal symptoms, headache, nausea, pulse irregularities, tremors, vomiting

## Special Nursing Considerations
## and Patient Education

- Monitor fluid levels, lithium serum levels (effective range: 1–1.5 mEq; *maintenance* range: 0.6–1.2 mEq), salt intake, weight.
- Arrange to have lithium levels drawn regularly (generally, daily until therapeutic dose established, then every 2 months).
- Be aware that
  - medication affects certain diagnostic tests (e.g., serum enzymes, glucose, magnesium).
- Teach patient to
  - notify physician for decrease in coordination, diarrhea, hand tremors, lethargy, muscle weakness, slurring of speech, vomiting.
  - not take any nonprescription medications without notifying physician.
  - take medication with milk or food to decrease gastric upset.
  - be cautious when driving or involved in potentially hazardous tasks.
  - use caution in hot weather and during strenuous exercise because they decrease patient's tolerance to lithium.

# Loxapine Succinate

**Brand Name**
Loxitane

**Actions**
Antipsychotic, tranquilizer

**Uses**
Psychotic disorders, schizophrenia

**Contraindications**
*Meds* Alcohol, CNS depressants
*Other* Children under 16, coma. *Use with caution:*
Brain tumor, cardiovascular dysfunction,
convulsive disorders, glaucoma, hypertension,
hypotension, intestinal obstruction, syncope,
tachycardia, urinary retention

**Interactions**
Anticholinergics, guanethidine

**Dose**
*Adult* PO: Initial dose: 10 mg bid; *maintenance* dose:
60–100 mg bid-qid; *maximum* dose: 250 mg/day

**Forms**
Capsules, concentrate, injection

**Adverse Effects**
Blurred vision, constipation, drowsiness, dry
mouth, extrapyramidal symptoms

## Special Nursing Considerations and Patient Education
- Dilute concentrate with water or juice (e.g., grapefruit, orange).
- Monitor for fine vermicular tongue movements (may indicate early tardive dyskinesia).
- Offer hard candy (regular or sugar-free) to relieve dry mouth.
- Teach patient
  - to be cautious when driving or involved in potentially hazardous tasks.
  - that medication may cause photosensitivity.
  - to notify physician for blurred vision, tremors, weakness.

# Maprotiline HCl

**Brand Name**
Ludiomil

**Actions**
Tetracyclic antidepressant; possible blockage of reuptake of norepinephrine at nerve endings. Onset evident in 3–7 days.

**Uses**
Depressive neurosis, manic-depression (depressive phase)

**Contraindications**
*Meds* Alcohol, MAO inhibitors
*Other* Children under 18, convulsive disorders. *Use with caution:* Closed-angle glaucoma; history of cardiovascular disease, convulsive disorders; MI or thyroid problems, increased intraocular pressure; urinary retention

**Interactions**
Anticholinergics, clonidine, CNS depressants, guanethidine, sympathomimetics, thyroid medication

**Dose**
*Adult* Initial dose: 75 mg/day; *maintenance* dose: 75–100 mg/day; *maximum* dose: inpatient 300 mg/day, outpatient 225 mg/day

**Forms**
Tablets

**Adverse Effects**
Blurred vision, constipation, convulsions, dizziness, drowsiness, dry mouth, insomnia, nervousness, tremors

**Special Nursing Considerations
and Patient Education**
- Use caution when administering to a patient with suicidal potential; ensure patient swallows dose.
- Offer hard candy (regular or sugar-free) to relieve dry mouth.
- Teach patient
  - to be cautious when driving or involved in potentially hazardous tasks.

# Meclizine HCl

**Brand Name**
Antivert, Bonine, Meclizine Hydrochloride

**Actions**
Antihistamine, antinausea; decreases sensitivity of CNS and inner ear to select stimuli. Onset evident in 1 hour.

**Uses**
Prevention of motion sickness

**Contraindications**
*Meds*  Alcohol, CNS depressants, MAO inhibitors
*Other*  Children, pregnancy. *Use with caution:* Allergy to antihistamines, bladder-neck or pyloro-duodenal obstruction, narrow-angle glaucoma, prostatic hypertrophy

**Interactions**
Amphetamines, antidepressants, atropine, hypnotics, narcotics, ototoxics, sedatives, tranquilizers

**Dose**
*Adult*  25–100 mg qd

**Forms**
Chewable and regular tablets

**Adverse Effects**
Blurred vision, drowsiness, dry mouth

## Special Nursing Considerations
## and Patient Education

- Offer hard candy (regular or sugar free) to relieve dry mouth.
- Be aware that
  - medication is most effective when administered 1 hour before departure.
- Teach patient
  - to be cautious when driving or involved in potentially hazardous tasks.

# Meclofenamate Sodium

**Brand Name**
Meclomen

**Actions**
Antirheumatic; hinders synthesis of prostaglandin

**Uses**
Osteoarthritis or rheumatoid arthritis

**Contraindications**
Allergic rhinitis, bronchospasm, children under 14, urticaria due to aspirin or nonsteroid inflammatory medications. *Use with caution:* History of upper GI disease

**Interactions**
Aspirin, CNS depressants, oral anticoagulants

**Dose**
*Adult* 200–400 mg in 3–4 divided doses; *maximum* dose: 400 mg/day

**Forms**
Capsules

**Adverse Effects**
Abdominal pain, anorexia, constipation, diarrhea, dizziness, flatulence, hepatitis, nausea, pyrosis, tarry stools, visual difficulties, vomiting

## Special Nursing Considerations
## and Patient Education
- Teach patient
  - to be cautious when driving or involved in potentially hazardous tasks.
  - to notify physician for abdominal pain, diarrhea, nausea, rash, tarry stools, vomiting.

# Mefenamic Acid

**Brand Name**
Ponstel

**Actions**
Analgesic, anti-inflammatory, antipyretic

**Uses**
Mild to moderate pain

**Contraindications**
Children under 14, chronic GI tract inflammation, ulceration. *Use with caution:* Asthma, diabetes, hepatic or renal dysfunction

**Interactions**
Aspirin, CNS depressants, oral anticoagulants

**Dose**
*Adult* Initial dose: 500 mg; then 250 mg q6h

**Forms**
Capsules

**Adverse Effects**
Confusion, diarrhea, dizziness, drowsiness, dysuria, eye irritation, flatulence, GI cramps, headache, hematuria, insomnia, nausea, nervousness, urticaria, vomiting

**Special Nursing Considerations
and Patient Education**
- Be aware that
  - treatment is usually no longer than 1 week.
- Teach patient to
  - be cautious when driving or involved in potentially hazardous tasks.
  - discontinue for diarrhea.
  - take medication with food to help decrease GI upset.

# Meperidine HCl

**Brand Name**
Demerol

**Actions**
Antispasmodic, CNS depressant (cortical, subcortical levels), narcotic analgesic. Onset evident in 15 minutes.

**Uses**
Preoperative medication, severe pain

**Contraindications**
*Meds* Alcohol, MAO inhibitors
*Other* Gallbladder or bile duct disorders, hepatic dysfunction, increased intracranial pressure. *Use with caution:* Addison's disease, cardiac dysrhythmias, epilepsy, glaucoma, head injuries, hypothyroidism, prostatic hypertrophy, renal dysfunction, respiratory impairment, urethral stricture

**Interactions**
Anticholinergics, antidepressants, CNS depressants, diuretics, hypnotics, narcotics, sedatives, skeletal muscle relaxants, tranquilizers

**Dose**
*Adult* PO: 50–150 mg q3–4h
*Peds* PO: 1 mg/kg q4h prn

**Forms**
Injection, tablets

## Adverse Effects

Dizziness, dry mouth, euphoria, headache, light-headedness, nausea, orthostatic hypotension, respiratory difficulty, syncope, tachycardia, vomiting

## Special Nursing Considerations
## and Patient Education

- Check blood pressure and respiratory rate prior to administration. Respirations should be at least 12/minute; BP per individual guidelines. Hold dose if minimum levels are not met.
- Offer hard candy (regular or sugar-free) to relieve dry mouth.
- Rotate injection sites.
- Teach patient to
  - avoid alcohol and other CNS depressants
  - be cautious when driving or involved in potentially hazardous tasks.
  - not smoke after receiving medications because of safety factor.
  - change position slowly to decrease hypotension.

# Mephenytoin

**Brand Name**
Mesantoin

**Actions**
Anticonvulsant

**Uses**
Epilepsy (focal, grand mal, jacksonian, psychomotor seizures), refractory to other medications

**Contraindications**
*Meds* Alcohol, CNS depressants
*Other* Hypersensitivity. *Use with caution:* Impaired hepatic function

**Interactions**
Isoniazid, oral anticoagulants, phenylbutazone, sulfonamides

**Dose**
*Adult* Individualized; initial dose: 50–100 mg/day, gradually increased; *maintenance* dose: 200–800 mg/day in divided doses
*Peds* Individualized; initial dose: 50–100 mg/day, gradually increased; *maintenance* dose: 3–15 mg/kg/day in 3 divided doses

**Forms**
Tablets

**Adverse Effects**
Blood dyscrasias, dizziness, drowiness, fever, insomnia, rash

## Special Nursing Considerations
## and Patient Education
- Supervise patient closely because of possibility of severe side effects.
- When discontinued, decrease dosage gradually.
- Be aware that
  - tolerance can develop.
  - that this medication is used only after safer anticonvulsants have been utilized.
- Teach patient
  - to be cautious when driving or involved in potentially hazardous tasks.
  - signs of an impending toxic reaction (e.g., ataxia, drowsiness, fever, mucus membrane hemorrhage, skin rash, sore throat).

# Meprobamate

**Brand Name**
Equanil, Meprospan, Miltown

**Actions**
Antianxiety, anticonvulsant, hypnotic, muscle relaxant, sedative

**Uses**
Anxiety, insomnia, tension

**Contraindications**
*Meds* Alcohol, CNS depressants
*Other* Acute intermittent porphyria, allergy to chemically related medications, children under 6 years. *Use with caution:* Epilepsy, hepatic or renal dysfunction

**Interactions**
Anticonvulsants, antidepressants, hypnotics, MAO inhibitors, oral anticoagulants, sedatives, tranquilizers

**Dose**
*Adult* PO: 400 mg tid–qid; *maximum* dose: 2.4 gm/day
*Peds* PO: Over 6 yr: initial dose, 100–200 mg bid–tid

**Forms**
Injection, suspension, sustained-release capsules, tablets

**Adverse Effects**
Blurred vision, dizziness, drowsiness, dysrhythmias, hypotension, paresthesia, slurring of speech, syncope, weakness

## Special Nursing Considerations and Patient Education

- Do not crush sustained-release capsules.
- Use caution when administering to a patient with suicidal potential; ensure patient swallows dose.
- Help patient to verbalize anxious feelings.
- Discontinue for ecchymosis, fever, hemorrhage, rash, sore throat.
- Be aware that
  - dependence is possible; when discontinued, decrease dosage gradually.
- Teach patient
  - to be cautious when driving or involved in potentially hazardous tasks.
  - to change position slowly since dizziness from hypotension may result in injury.
  - to decrease caffeine intake because of its stimulant effect.

# Meprobamate/Tridihexethyl Chloride

## Brand Name
Milpath, Pathibamate

## Actions
Anticholinergic, antimuscarinic, antispasmodic, parasympatholytic; competes with acetylcholine for postganglionic fiber receptors (muscarinic)

## Uses
Acute entero- or mucous colitis, functional GI disturbances, irritable or spastic colon disorders

## Contraindications
*Meds* MAO inhibitors
*Other* Adhesions between iris and lens, asthma, children under 12, hepatic or renal impairment, hiatal hernia associated with reflex esophagitis, intestinal atony, myasthenia gravis, narrow-angle glaucoma, obstructive disease of GI or urinary tract, severe ulcerative colitis. *Use with caution:* Angina pectoris, chronic bronchitis, coronary disease, hiatal hernia, open-angle glaucoma, prostatic hypertrophy

## Interactions
Antacids, antihistamines, atropine-like medications, haloperidol, meperidine, methylphenidate, nitrates, nitrites, orphenadrine, phenothiazines, pilocarpine, tricyclic antidepressants

## Dose
*Adult* PO: 25–50 mg 3–4x/day; parenteral: 10–20 mg q6h

## Forms
Injection, coated tablets, tablets

## Adverse Effects
Blurred vision, constipation, drowsiness, eye pain, flushing, headaches, hypotension, urinary hesitancy

## Special Nursing Considerations and Patient Education
- Administer oral forms before meals and at hs.
- Teach patient
  - to use caution when driving or involved in potentially hazardous tasks.
  - to not take any nonprescription cough or hay fever medications.
  - if taking antacids, to do so several hours apart from this medication.
  - to notify physician for flushing, eye pain, rash
  - to use caution in hot weather and during strenuous exercise because these situations potentiate the medication's hypotensive effects.

# Metaraminol Bitartrate

**Brand Name**
  Aramine

**Actions**
  Cardiac stimulant, peripheral vasoconstrictor,
  vasopressor; stimulates norepinephrine release
  from tissues, plus direct alpha stimulation. Onset
  evident: IM 10 minutes; IV 1–2 minutes; SC 5–20
  minutes

**Uses**
  Hypotension, shock

**Contraindications**
  Cyclopropane, halothane. *Use with caution:*
  Cardiac disease, cirrhosis, diabetes, digitalized
  patients, hypertension, hyperthyroidism, malaria

**Interactions**
  Digitalis, guanethidine, MAO inhibitors, oxytocics,
  reserpine, tricyclic antidepressants

**Dose**
*Adult*  IM/SC: 2–10 mg; IV: 0.05–5 mg; infusion:
         15–100 mg in 500 cc of titrate
*Peds*   IM/SC: 0.1 mg/kg; IV: 0.4 mg/kg; infusion: 0.4
         mg/kg

**Forms**
  Injection

**Adverse Effects**
  Dysrhythmias, headache, hyperglycemia,
  hypertension, nausea, palpitations, tissue
  necrosis, tremors, vomiting

## Special Nursing Considerations and Patient Education

- Protect medication from heat and direct light.
- Check blood pressure before administration; compare to parameters for each patient and take appropriate action as necessary.
- Correct blood volume prior to administration.
- Monitor blood pressure (infusion: q5min until stable, then q15min), CVP, injection sites, I&O.
- When discontinued, decrease dosage gradually to avoid withdrawal problems.

# Methadone HCl

## Brand Name
Dolophine Hydrochloride

## Actions
Analgesic, antitussive. Onset evident: PO 30–60 minutes; IV: 10–15 minutes.

## Uses
Heroin withdrawal, relief of severe pain

## Contraindications
*Meds* Alcohol

*Other* Children, hepatic disease (IV usage). *Use with caution:* Addison's disease, asthma, cardiac dysrhythmias, chronic ulcerative colitis, gallbladder disease, hepatic or renal impairment, hypothyroidism, prostatic hypertrophy, respiratory disease, urethral stricture

## Interactions
Anticholinergics, antidepressants, CNS depressants, diuretics, hypnotics, narcotics, sedatives, skeletal muscle relaxants, tranquilizers

## Dose
*Adult* PO: Pain: individualized; usually 2.5–10 mg q3–4h; *withdrawal* dose: 20–40 mg/day in divided doses; *maintenance* dose: 40–120 mg or higher qd

## Forms
Injection, syrup, tablets

## Adverse Effects

Constipation, dizziness, drowsiness, dry mouth, euphoria, impotence, nausea, orthostatic hypotension, vomiting

## Special Nursing Considerations and Patient Education

- Protect medication from direct light.
- Offer hard candy (regular or sugar-free) to relieve dry mouth.
- Be aware that
  - medication is cumulative.
  - dependence is possible; when discontinued, decrease dosage gradually.
- Teach patient
  - to be cautious when driving or involved in potentially hazardous tasks.
  - to change position slowly to decrease hypotension.

# Methicillin Sodium

**Brand Name**
Staphcillin

**Actions**
Antibiotic, anti-infective, bactericidal

**Uses**
Bacterial endocarditis, enterocolitis, infections
that are penicillin G and staphylococcus resistant,
osteomyelitis, septicemia

**Contraindications**
Hypersensitivity to penicillins or cephalosporins.
*Use with caution*: Renal dysfunction

**Interactions**
Erythromycin, probenecid, tetracycline

**Dose**
*Adult* IM: 1 gm q4–6h; IV: 1 gm q6h
*Peds* 25 mg/kg q6h

**Forms**
Injection, piggyback injection

**Adverse Effects**
Bone-marrow depression, interstitial nephritis, pain
at injection site, penicillin-type allergy

## Special Nursing Considerations and Patient Education

- Adhere to specific directions for IV solution compatibility and reconstitution of medication.
- Do not mix with any other medications in an IV solution or syringe.
- Inject IM dose deep into gluteal muscle.
- Rotate injection sites; monitor for inflammation.
- Determine if patient has had this medication before. If not, monitor patient's reaction carefully.
- Keep out-patient client in clinic/office for 30 minutes after receiving injection.
- Be aware that
  - medication is sensitive to heat.
  - cross-resistance to cephalosporin medication may develop.

# Methohexital Sodium

**Brand Name**
Brevital

**Actions**
Anesthetic

**Uses**
Hypnotic induction, surgery

**Contraindications**
*Meds* Alcohol, CNS depressants
*Other* Status asthmaticus, porphyria. *Use with caution:* Addison's disease, anemia, cardiovascular disease, hepatic or renal dysfunction, hypertension, increased intracranial pressure or serum urea, myasthenia gravis, myxedema

**Interactions**
Acid solutions

**Dose**
*Adult* Individualized; initial dose: 50–120 mg IV; *maintenance* dose: 20–40 mg q4–7min

**Forms**
Injection

**Adverse Effects**
Abnormal muscle movements, bronchospasm, dysrhythmias, hiccoughs, laryngospasm, myocardial or respiratory depression, sneezing

**Special Nursing Considerations
and Patient Education**
- Maintain a patent airway.
- Do not mix any other medications in infusion solution.
- Do not use bacteriostatic diluents.
- Monitor vital signs.
- Keep endotracheal intubation, resuscitation equipment, and oxygen readily available.

# Methyldopa

**Brand Name**
  Aldomet

**Actions**
  Stimulates alpha-adrenergic receptors (central inhibiting). Onset evident: PO 6-12 hours; IV 4-6 hours.

**Uses**
  Complicated, renal hypertension; hypertension

**Contraindications**
*Meds*  Alcohol, CNS depressants, MAO inhibitors, tricyclic antidepressants
*Other*  History of depression, pheochromocytoma. *Use with caution:* Bilateral cerebrovascular disease, history of hepatic disease, renal impairment

**Interactions**
  Amphetamines, antihypertensives, haloperidol

**Dose**
*Adult*  PO: 250 mg bid-tid x3/day; *maintenance* dose: 500 mg-2 gm/day in divided doses
*Peds*  PO: 10-65 mg/kg/day in 2-4 divided doses

**Forms**
  Injection (-pate hydrochloride), tablets

**Adverse Effects**
  Bradycardia, depression, diarrhea, dizziness, edema, headache, hepatitis, nausea, orthostatic hypotension, positive direct Coombs' test, sedation, vomiting, weakness

## Special Nursing Considerations and Patient Education

- Adjust dosage at 2-day intervals in order to reach a maintenance dosage.
- When changing medication to or from other antihypertensives, do so gradually.
- Monitor blood pressure, I&O, neurologic status, renal function, weight.
- Be aware that
  - tolerance can develop if patient is not on a diuretic.
- Teach patient
  - that hot baths or showers may aggravate hypotension.
  - to change position slowly to decrease hypotension.
  - that medication may cause tongue to appear black or turn urine blue/dark.
  - that medication may cause photosensitivity.
  - to be cautious when driving or involved in potentially hazardous tasks.
  - to use caution during strenuous exercise as it may increase orthostatic hypotension.
  - to notify physician for fever, urine darkening.

# Methylphenidate HCl

**Brand Name**
Ritalin Hydrochloride

**Actions**
CNS stimulant; affects the cerebral cortex and subcortical structures

**Uses**
Attention-deficit disorders, hyperkinesis, mild depression, narcolepsy, withdrawn senile behavior

**Contraindications**
*Meds* MAO inhibitors, pressors
*Other* Agitation, anxiety, children under 6, glaucoma, severe depression, tension. *Use with caution:* Emotional instability, epilepsy, history of alcoholism or drug dependence, hypertension, psychosis

**Interactions**
Anticholinergics, anticoagulants, anticonvulsants, desipramine, guanethidine, imipramine, phenobarbital, phenytoin, primadone, tricyclic antidepressants

**Dose**
*Adult* PO: 20–30 mg/day in 2–3 divided doses
*Peds* PO: 5 mg before breakfast or lunch; increased by 5–10 mg weekly; *maximum* dose: 60 mg/day

**Forms**
Injection, tablets

**Adverse Effects**
Angina, anorexia, blurred vision, dizziness, dyskinesia, headache, insomnia, nervousness, tachycardia, weight loss

## Special Nursing Considerations
## and Patient Education
- Administer medication 30–45 minutes before meals.
- Monitor blood pressure, pulse, weight.
- In children, discontinue if there is no evidence of improvement within one month; long-term therapy may impair growth.
- If patient has insomnia, administer last dose by 6:00 P.M.
- Be aware that
  - dependence is possible; when discontinued, gradually decrease dosage.
  - tolerance can develop.
- Teach patient
  - to be cautious when driving or involved in potentially hazardous tasks.

# Methyprylon

**Brand Name**
Noludar

**Actions**
CNS depressant, hypnotic, sedative. Onset evident in 30 minutes.

**Uses**
Insomnia

**Contraindications**
Alcohol, CNS depressants. *Use with caution:* Hepatic or renal disease, porphyria

**Interactions**
Antihistamines, barbiturates, hypnotics, MAO inhibitors, phenothiazines, sedatives, tranquilizers, tricyclic antidepressants

**Dose**
*Adult*  200–400 mg/day
*Peds*  Initial dose: 50 mg/day; may increase up to 200 mg/day

**Forms**
Capsules, elixir, tablets

**Adverse Effects**
Diarrhea, dizziness, excitability, headache, morning drowsiness, nausea, rash, vomiting

## Special Nursing Considerations and Patient Education
- Protect medication from direct light.
- Use caution when administering to a patient with suicidal potential; ensure patient swallows dose.
- For use as a hypnotic, administer 15 minutes before going to bed.
- Be aware that
  - medication may be habit-forming; when discontinued, decrease dosage gradually.
- Teach patient
  - to be cautious when driving or involved in potentially hazardous tasks.

# Metolazone

**Brand Name**
Diulo, Zaroxlyn

**Actions**
Antihypertensive, thiazide diuretic

**Uses**
Edema, hypertension

**Contraindications**
*Meds* Hypersensitivity to sulfa drugs
*Other* Anuria, arteriosclerosis, hepatic and pre-
hepatic coma, hepatic cirrhosis, renal function
impairment. *Use with caution:* Diabetes,
hypercalcemia, hyperuricemia, lupus
erythematosus, pancreatitis, sympathectomy

**Interactions**
ACTH, corticosteroids, lithium, oral hypoglycemics

**Dose**
*Adult* Edema: 5–20 mg qd; hypertension: 2.5–5 mg qd

**Forms**
Tablets

**Adverse Effects**
Bloating, chest pain, chills, diarrhea, dizziness, dry
mouth, hypokalemia, muscle cramps, nausea,
palpitations, pulse irregularities, thirst

## Special Nursing Considerations and Patient Education
- Administer in a single dose in morning.
- Monitor blood pressure, serum potassium.
- Offer hard candy (regular or sugar-free) to relieve dry mouth.
- Teach patient
  - that medication may cause photosensitivity.
  - to be cautious when driving or involved in potentially hazardous tasks.

# Metoprolol Tartrate

**Brand Name**
 Lopressor

**Actions**
 Antihypertensive; stops access of catecholamine
 to neurotransmitters to cardiac muscle beta₁
 receptors

**Uses**
 Hypertension

**Contraindications**
*Meds* MAO inhibitors
*Other* Cardiogenic shock, children, overt cardiac
 failure, sinus bradycardia. *Use with caution:*
 Angina, bronchospastic disease, cardiac
 dysfunction, congestive heart failure, diabetes,
 hepatic or renal impairment, thyrotoxicosis

**Interactions**
 Digitalis, diuretics, dobutamine, dopamine,
 isoproterenol, norepinephrine bitartrate, reserpine

**Dose**
*Adult* Individualized; initial dose: 50 mg bid adjusted
 weekly; *maintenance* dose: 100 mg bid

**Forms**
 Tablets

**Adverse Effects**
 Bradycardia, congestive heart failure, constipation,
 depression, diarrhea, disorientation, dizziness,
 dyspepsia, fatigue, hallucinations, hypotension,
 nausea, palpitations, shortness of breath,
 wheezing

**Special Nursing Considerations
and Patient Education**
- Administer medication before meals to enhance absorption.
- Monitor blood pressure, neurologic status, renal function.
- Teach patient to
  - be cautious when driving or involved in potentially hazardous tasks.
  - not discontinue without notifying physician.

# Metronidazole

**Brand Name**
Flagyl

**Actions**
Amebicide, antiprotozoan, systemic trichomonacide; hinders release of hydrogen for metabolic use in susceptible microorganisms

**Uses**
Chagas disease, giardiasis, hepatic or luminal form of *Entamoeba histolytica*, leishmaniasis

**Contraindications**
*Meds* Alcohol
*Other* Blood dyscrasias, CNS organic disease. *Use with caution:* Diabetes

**Interactions**
Oral anticoagulants

**Dose**
*Adult* PO: 250 mg tid x 7 days; IV: 15 mg/kg over 1 hr (load), then 7.5 mg/kg q6h
*Peds* PO: 35–50 mg/kg/day in 3 divided doses x 10 days

**Forms**
Injection, tablets

**Adverse Effects**
Abdominal cramps, anorexia, ataxia, constipation, diarrhea, dry mouth, headache, metallic taste, nausea, paresthesia, rash, seizures, vomiting

**Special Nursing Considerations
and Patient Education**
- Protect medication from light.
- Arrange treatment for sexual partner(s).
- Offer hard candy (regular or sugar-free) to relieve dry mouth.
- Teach patient
  - that medication may cause a metallic taste in mouth or dark brown urine.
  - to be cautious when driving or involved in potentially hazardous tasks.
  - to notify physician if numbness in feet and/or hands occurs.

# Minocycline HCl

**Brand Name**
Minocin

**Actions**
Antiamebic, antibacterial, antibiotic, anti-infective; hinders synthesis of protein in susceptible microorganisms

**Uses**
Granuloma inguinale, lymphogranuloma, mycoplasma, ornithosis, psittacosis, rickettsial disease, spirochetal relapsing fever

**Contraindications**
*Meds* Antacids, antidiarrheal suspensions, dairy products, penicillins
*Other* Allergy to tetracycline, children under 8 years, renal insufficiency. *Use with caution:* Hepatic or renal dysfunction, lupus erythematosus

**Interactions**
Barbiturates, carbaniazepine, oral anticoagulants, phenytoin, sodium bicarbonate

**Dose**
*Adult* PO: Initial dose 200 mg, then 100–200 mg q12h
*Peds* PO: Over 8 yr: initial dose 4 mg/kg, then 2 mg/kg q12h

**Forms**
Capsules, injection, syrup, tablets

**Adverse Effects**
Ataxia, dizziness, flatulence, light-headedness, nausea, vertigo, vomiting, weakness

**Special Nursing Considerations
and Patient Education**
- Protect medication from light.
- Check expiration date to avoid severe reactions.
- Administer parenterally *only* if oral route is not tolerated.
- Monitor I&O.
- Teach patient
  - to continue treatment for beta-hemolytic group A streptococci infections for 10 days.
  - to take drug before meals or 2 hours after meals, to not take within an hour of hs.
  - to take with a full glass of water. Do not take with antacids, antidiarrheal suspensions, or dairy products.
  - that medication may cause photosensitivity.
  - to be cautious when driving or involved in potentially hazardous tasks.

# Minoxidil

**Brand Name**
Loniten

**Actions**
Antihypertensive; relaxation and vasodilation of arteriolar muscle

**Uses**
Hypertension that is not manageable with maximum therapeutic dosage of two antihypertensives plus a diuretic

**Contraindications**
Pheochromocytoma. *Use with caution:* Dialysis, malignant hypertension, renal failure

**Interactions**
Guanethidine

**Dose**
*Adult* 10–40 mg/day; *maximum* dose: 100 mg/day
*Peds* 0.2–1 mg/kg/day; *maximum* dose: 50 mg/day

**Forms**
Tablets

**Adverse Effects**
Arm, chest, and shoulder pain; breast tenderness; dizziness; dyspepsia; hypertrichosis; orthostatic hypotension; pericardial effusion; respiratory difficulty; salt and water retention; tachycardia (while resting); weight gain

## Special Nursing Considerations
## and Patient Education

- Monitor blood pressure, electrolytes, fluids, neurologic status, renal function, weight.
- Be aware that
  - this drug is usually administered with a beta-adrenergic blocking agent and a diuretic.
  - this medication controls blood pressure slowly.
- Teach patient
  - that medication may cause darkening and growth of fine body hair.
  - to notify physician for dizziness; dyspepsia; faintness; *new* pain in arm, chest, shoulder; increase in resting pulse over 20 beats; increase in respiratory difficulty; rapid weight gain over 5 pounds.

# Molindone HCl

**Brand Name**
Moban

**Actions**
Antipsychotic, tranquilizer; acts on ascending reticular activating system; onset time: 1.5 hours peak plasma level, duration of single dose 24–36 hours

**Uses**
Schizophrenia

**Contraindications**
*Meds* Alcohol, CNS depressants
*Other* Children under 12, coma. *Use with caution:* Brain tumors, convulsive disorders, intestinal obstructions

**Interactions**
Atropine, barbiturates, guanethidine, narcotics

**Dose**
*Adult* Initial dose: 50–75 mg/day; increase to 100 mg/day over 3–4 days; *maintenance* dose: 20–225 mg/day
*Peds* Adolescent: same as adult

**Forms**
Concentrated solution, tablets

**Adverse Effects**
Blurred vision, constipation, drowsiness, dry mouth, extrapyramidal symptoms, urinary retention

## Special Nursing Considerations and Patient Education

- Monitor for fine vermicular tongue movements (may indicate early tardive dyskinesia).
- Offer hard candy (regular or sugar-free) to relieve dry mouth.
- Teach patient
  - to be cautious when driving or involved in potentially hazardous tasks.
  - to notify physician of tremors, vision impairment, weakness.

# Morphine Sulfate

**Brand Name**
Morphine

**Actions**
Analgesic; impedes pain impulses at subcortical level. Onset evident in 20 minutes.

**Uses**
Burns, pain, shock

**Contraindications**
Alcohol, CNS depressants. *Use with caution:* Acute alcoholism, Addison's disease, atrial flutter, cardiac dysrhythmias, convulsive disorders, gallbladder disease, head injuries, hepatic or renal dysfunction, hypotension, hypothyroidism, myxedema, prostatic hypertrophy, toxic psychosis

**Interactions**
Anesthetics, anticholinergics, antihistamines, benzodiazepines, MAO inhibitors, papaverine, phenothiazines, skeletal muscle relaxants, tricyclic antidepressants

**Dose**
*Adult*  PO: 5–15 mg q4h
*Peds*  PO: 0.1–0.2 mg/kg/dose; *maximum* dose: 15 mg/single dose

**Forms**
Atropine injection, injection, tablets

**Adverse Effects**
Anorexia, constipation, drowsiness, dysphoria, euphoria, hypotension, nausea, respiratory depression, spasm of biliary tract, tremors, vomiting, weakness

**Special Nursing Considerations
and Patient Education**
- Protect medication from direct light.
- If respirations are less than 10–12, hold medication.
- When discontinued, decrease dose gradually.
- Monitor bowel pattern, I&O, vital signs.
- Be aware that
  - patient may become addicted to medication.
- Teach (hospital) patient to
  - not smoke or walk without assistance due to the presence of possible side effects.
  - change position slowly to decrease hypotension.

# Nalorphine Hydrochloride

**Brand Name**
Nalline Hydrochloride

**Actions**
Antidote for narcotic respiratory depression. Onset evident in 1–2 minutes.

**Uses**
Poisoning by morphine-related analgesics

**Contraindications**
Drug abuse, narcotic addiction. *Use with caution:* Non-narcotic respiratory depression

**Interactions**
None

**Dose**
*Adult* 2–10 mg up to 3 doses
*Peds* 0.1 mg/kg/dose; *maximum* dose: 3 doses

**Forms**
Injection

**Adverse Effects**
Bradycardia, drowsiness, headache, hypotension, lethargy, nausea, respiratory depression, tremors, vomiting

**Special Nursing Considerations
and Patient Education**
- Protect medication from direct light.
- Monitor vital signs throughout treatment.

# Naloxone Hydrochloride

**Brand Name**
Narcan

**Actions**
Narcotic antagonist for receptor sites in CNS.
Onset evident in 2 minutes (IV).

**Uses**
Narcotic or respiratory depression, opiate
overdosage

**Contraindications**
Hypersensitivity

**Interactions**
None

**Dose**
*Adult* 0.4 mg/dose q2–3min; may have 2–3 doses
*Peds* 0.01 mg/kg/dose q2–3min; may have 2–3 doses

**Forms**
Injection

**Adverse Effects**
Drowsiness, hypertension, hyperventilation,
nausea, tachycardia, tremors, vomiting

**Special Nursing Considerations
and Patient Education**
- Protect medication from direct light.
- Monitor vital signs.
- Be aware that
    - dependence is possible; when discontinued,
      decrease dosage gradually.
    - failure of the patient to respond may indicate
      that the respiratory depression is not only a
      result from opiate intoxication.

# Neostigmine

**Brand Name**
Prostigmin Bromide

**Actions**
Cholinergic, muscarinic, nicotinic; inhibits cholinergic-acetylcholinesterase

**Uses**
Amenorrhea, bowel ileus, closed- or open-angle glaucoma, megacolon, myasthenia gravis, pregnancy testing, tubocurarine poisoning, urinary retention

**Contraindications**
*Meds* Atropine, mecamylamine
*Other* Mechanical-intestinal or urinary obstruction.
   *Use caution:* Bronchial asthma

**Interactions**
Aminoglycosides

**Dose**
*Adult* PO: 15–30 mg tid–qid, gradually increased until desired response achieved; *maintenance* dose: 15–375 mg/day
*Peds* PO: 7.5–15 mg tid–qid

**Forms**
Methylsulfate injection, Bromide tablets

**Adverse Effects**
Abdominal cramps, diaphoresis, diarrhea, diplopia, hypotension, nausea, sneezing, urinary urgency, vomiting

## Special Nursing Considerations
## and Patient Education
- Take pulse before administering; should be over 80 beats/minute.
- Have atropine available in case of overdose.
- Keep accurate records of patient's responses to dosages.
- Notify physician for indications of cholinergic crisis (e.g., weakness 1 hour after treatment), or myasthenic crisis (weakness 3 hours after treatment).
- Teach patient
  - to avoid fatigue.

# Nitroglycerin

**Brand Name**
Nitro-Bid, Nitrol, Nitrostat

**Actions**
Vasodilator; relaxation of vascular smooth muscle. Onset evident in 1–5 minutes.

**Uses**
Angina pectoris

**Contraindications**
*Meds* Alcohol
*Other* Anemia, children, glaucoma, hypersensitivity to vasodilators, hyperthyroid, increased intracranial pressure, MI, tendency to hypotension

**Interactions**
Antihypertensives

**Dose**
*Adult* Individualized; PO: 2.5–6.5 mg q8–12h; sublingual: 0.4–0.6 mg prn; IV: 5–20 mcg/min

**Forms**
Injection, ointment, prolonged-action and sublingual tablets, sustained-release capsules

**Adverse Effects**
Dizziness, flushing, headache, nausea, palpitations, postural hypotension, tachycardia, vomiting

## Special Nursing Considerations and Patient Education

- Do not crush prolonged-action or sustained-release forms.
- When applying ointment, do not rub; rotate sites.
- When discontinued, decrease dosage and frequency over 4–6 weeks.
- Repeat dose if pain is not relieved in 5–10 minutes; consult physician if pain is not relieved in 15–20 minutes.
- Keep medication in original container; do not store with cotton.
- Do not use medication if it is older than 60 days.
- Be aware that
  - tolerance can develop.
  - medication is unstable; protect from air, heat, light, moisture.
- Teach patient to
  - change position slowly to decrease hypotension.
  - decrease smoking; be cautious in cold weather, during strenuous exercise, or with increased stress because these may cause increased episodes of angina pectoris.
  - not swallow sublingual tablets.
  - notify physician for blurred vision, dry mouth.

# Norepinephrine Bitartrate

**Brand Name**
  Levophed

**Actions**
  Peripheral vasoconstrictor, sympathomimetic,
  vasopressor; activates alpha and beta receptors

**Uses**
  Cardiogenic shock, hypotension

**Contraindications**
*Meds*  Cyclopropane anesthesia
*Other*  Mesenteric thrombosis

**Interactions**
  MAO inhibitors, tricyclic antidepressants

**Dose**
*Adult*  2–8 cc of 0.2% in 1 liter of 5% dextrose,
      infused at 2–4 mcg/minute
*Peds*  1 cc of 0.2% in 250 cc of 5% dextrose

**Forms**
  Injection

**Adverse Effects**
  Anxiety, dizziness, headache, hypertension, pallor,
  reflex bradycardia, respiratory difficulty

## Special Nursing Considerations and Patient Education

- Protect medication from direct light.
- Discard solution if brown.
- Correct existing hypovolemia prior to administering medication.
- Utilize large veins (avoid ankle, hand, and leg veins) to decrease risk of necrosis.
- Maintain patient's hydration.
- When discontinued, decrease dosage gradually.
- Monitor blood pressure (q2 minutes initially, then q5 minutes until 80–100 systolic) extremities (color and temperature), I&O, mental status.
- Ensure that IV does not infiltrate because of high risk of tissue damage.

# Nystatin

**Brand Name**
Mycostatin, Nilstat

**Actions**
Antibiotic, antifungal; causes leakage of essential components through walls of susceptible organisms

**Uses**
Candida albicans infections

**Contraindications**
Hypersensitivity

**Interactions**
None

**Dose**
*Adult* PO: 500,000–1,000,000 U tid
*Peds* PO: 100,000–600,000 U qid

**Forms**
Cream, ointment, powder, suspension, tablets, vaginal suppositories and tablets

**Adverse Effects**
Diarrhea, GI distress, nausea, vomiting

## Special Nursing Considerations and Patient Education

- Avoid contact with drugs by hands.
- Protect liquid form from heat and light; use within 1 week.
- Do not mix suspensions in foods.
- Give infants ½ of a dose in each side of mouth, to be retained as long as possible.
- Teach patient
  - to continue vaginal tablets when menstruating.
  - to continue treatment at least 48 hours after symptoms are gone.
  - to maintain good personal hygiene.

# Oxazepam

**Brand Name**
  Serax

**Actions**
  Antianxiety, hypnotic, sedative, tranquilizer. Onset evident in 1-2 hours.

**Uses**
  Acute alcohol withdrawal, anxiety, insomnia

**Contraindications**
*Meds*  Alcohol, CNS depressants
*Other*  Acute narrow-angle glaucoma, children, psychosis. *Use with caution:* Allergy to chemically related medications, epilepsy, hepatic or renal impairment, pulmonary disease

**Interactions**
  Antihistamines, barbiturates, cimetidine, MAO inhibitors, narcotics, phenothiazines, tricyclic antidepressants

**Dose**
*Adult*  10-30 mg tid-qid

**Forms**
  Capsules, tablets

**Adverse Effects**
  Ataxia, drowsiness, edema, euphoria, hypotension, lethargy, speech slurring, tremors

## Special Nursing Considerations
## and Patient Education
- Protect medication from direct light.
- Encourage patient to verbalize feelings of anxiety.
- Be aware that
  - medication can be addictive; when discontinued, decrease dosage gradually.
- Teach patient to
  - be cautious when driving or involved in potentially hazardous tasks.
  - notify physician for ecchymosis, eye pain, fever, hemorrhage, sore throat.

# Oxtriphylline

**Brand Name**
 Choledyl

**Actions**
 Bronchodilator

**Uses**
 Acute bronchial asthma, reversible bronchospasm

**Contraindications**
 Angina, coronary artery disease, hypotension. *Use
 with caution:* Acute MI, cardiovascular disease,
 congestive heart failure, glaucoma, hepatic or
 renal disease, hyperthyroidism, hypoxemia, peptic
 ulcer, porphyria, prostatic hypertrophy

**Interactions**
 Allopurinol, cimetidine, digitalis, erythromycin,
 furosemide, lincomycin, lithium carbonate, oral
 anticoagulants, phenobarbital, phenytoin,
 propranolol

**Dose**
*Adult* 100–200 mg qid
*Peds* 2–12 yr: 15 mg/kg/day in 4 divided doses

**Forms**
 Elixir, pediatric syrup, tablets

**Adverse Effects**
 Diarrhea, dizziness, gastric upset, headache,
 insomnia, irritability, nausea, vomiting

**Special Nursing Considerations
and Patient Education**
- Protect medication from heat and light.
- Administer after meals and at hs.
- Teach patient
  - to decrease smoking because it reduces
    medication's effectiveness.

# Oxymorphone Hydrochloride

**Brand Name**
Numorphan

**Actions**
Narcotic analgesic. Onset evident: SC 5–8 minutes; suppositories 15–30 minutes.

**Uses**
Acute vascular occlusion, burns, moderate to severe pain from biliary spasm, neoplastic disease, neurologic diseases, trauma

**Contraindications**
*Meds* Alcohol, CNS depressants
*Other* Acute undiagnosed abdominal conditions, Addison's disease, alcoholism, bronchial asthma, children, chronic pulmonary disease, convulsive disorder, hypothyroidism, increased intracranial pressure, pancreatitis, prostatic hypertrophy, pulmonary edema. *Use with caution:* Cardiac dysrhythmias, cardiovascular disease, cor pulmonale, emphysema, kypho-scoliosis, psychosis, severe obesity

**Interactions**
Anesthetics, anticholinergics, antihistamines, benzodiazepines, MAO inhibitors, papaverine, phenothiazines, skeletal muscle relaxants, tricyclic antidepressants

**Dose**
*Adult* IM/SC: 1–1.5 mg q4–6h

**Forms**
Injection, suppositories

## Adverse Effects

Bradycardia, constipation, dizziness, euphoria, nausea, vomiting

## Special Nursing Considerations and Patient Education

- Protect medication from light.
- Store suppositories in refrigerator.
- Monitor bowel movements, I&O, vital signs.
- Hold medications if respirations are less than 10–12.
- Be aware that
  - dependence is possible; when discontinued, decrease dosage gradually.
  - that medication can be toxic.
- Teach patient
  - to be cautious when driving or involved in potentially hazardous tasks.
  - to walk with assistance and to not smoke because of medication's side effects.

# Oxytocin

## Brand Name
Pitocin, Syntocinon

## Actions
Hormone; increases permeability of sodium ions in uterine cells leading to increased numbers of contracting myofibrils. Onset evident: buccal 30 minutes; IM 3–7 minutes; IV 1 minute.

## Uses
Labor induction, uterine hemorrhage or inertia

## Contraindications
Amniotic fluid embolism, cephalopelvic disproportion, children, fetal distress or malpresentation, first stage labor, hyper- or hypotonic uterine contractions, severe medical conditions or toxemia, thromboplastin predisposition, uterine overdistention

## Interactions
None

## Dose
*Adult*  Individualized; 10–40 U in 1,000 cc of 5% dextrose

## Forms
Citrate buccal tablets; synthetic injection and nasal spray

## Adverse Effects
*Fetus*  Bradycardia, death, dysrhythmias, hypoxia, internal hemorrhage

*Mother*  Convulsions, dysrhythmias, hypertensive crisis, hypotension, pelvic hematoma, tetanic uterine contractions, uterine rupture

**Special Nursing Considerations
and Patient Education**
- Administer only 1 route at a time.
- Do not give IV in undiluted form or in high concentration.
- Administer medication exactly as directed.
- Monitor patient constantly for duration and frequency of contractions, fetal heart rate and tone, I&O, vital signs.
- Report contractions that are excessively long (over 90 seconds) or strong (50 mm Hg).

# Papaverine HCl

**Brand Name**
Cerebid, Cerespan, Pavabid

**Actions**
Antispasmodic, peripheral vasodilator; relaxes peripheral blood vessels. Onset evident in 30–60 minutes.

**Uses**
Cerebral, myocardial, or peripheral ischemia; circulatory disorders (blood vessel spasm)

**Contraindications**
*Meds* Alcohol
*Other* Children, complete A-V block, smoking. *Use with caution:* Circulatory dysfunction, coronary insufficiency, CVA, glaucoma, MI

**Dose**
*Adult* Individualized; PO: 100–300 mg 3–5x/day (sustained-release forms) or 150 mg q12h

**Forms**
Injection, long-acting capsules, tablets

**Adverse Effects**
Anorexia, constipation, diarrhea, dizziness, flushing, headache, nausea, sedation, sweating, vomiting

## Special Nursing Considerations and Patient Education

- Protect medication from heat and light.
- Do not mix medication with Ringer's Lactate.
- Do not crush long-acting capsules.
- Administer IV dose over 1–2 minutes.
- Monitor blood pressure, pulse, respirations (parenteral use).
- Teach patient
  - to be cautious when driving or involved in potentially hazardous tasks.
  - to use caution during exercise to avoid dizziness.

# Penicillin G

**Brand Name**
Bicillin

**Actions**
Antibacterial, antibiotic, anti-infective

**Uses**
Infections due to gram positive bacteria

**Contraindications**
Hypersensitivity to penicillin

**Interactions**
Aspirin, erythromycin, oral contraceptives or neomycin, phenylbutazone, probenecid, tetracycline

**Dose**
*Adult* IV: 400,000–600,000 U q4-6h
PO: 400,000–500,000 q6-8h
*Peds* Under 12 yr: 25,000–90,000 U/kg PO in 3–6 divided doses/day

**Forms**
Injection, suspension, tablets

**Adverse Effects**
Dermatitis, erythema, fever, interstitial nephritis, neurotoxicities, pruritus, urticaria

## Special Nursing Considerations
## and Patient Education
- Store oral liquid forms in refrigerator and discard after 14 days.
- Utilize a 20 gauge needle for doses over 300,000 U; use a 22 gauge needle for doses 300,000 or less.
- Shake vial after adding diluent to powder.
- Administer IM dose deep into muscle; do not massage; rotate sites.
- Monitor patient for allergic reaction if receiving this medication for first time; keep in out-patient clinic for 30 minutes after receiving injection.

# Penicillin V Potassium

**Brand Name**
Pen-Vee K, V-Cillin K

**Actions**
Antibiotic, anti-infective; hinders ability of bacteria to synthesize cell walls

**Uses**
Infections (gonococci, pneumococci, staphylococci, streptococci), rheumatic fever, surgery

**Contraindications**
Allergy to any penicillin. *Use with caution:* Allergy to cephalosporins, general allergies

**Interactions**
Chloramphenicol, erythromycin, neomycin, paromomycin, tetracycline, troleandomycin

**Dose**
*Adult* 250–500 mg tid–qid
*Peds* 15–50 mg/kg in 3–6 divided doses

**Forms**
Capsules, pediatric drops or suspension, solution, suspension, tablets

**Adverse Effects**
Anemia, black "hairy" tongue, diarrhea, nausea, superinfections, vomiting

## Special Nursing Considerations and Patient Education

- Administer one hour before or two hours after meals.
- Have out-patient stay for 30 minutes after receiving medication in case of allergic reaction.
- Teach patient
  - that medication may cause tongue to darken.
  - to complete full course of therapy.

# Pentaerythritol Tetranitrate

**Brand Name**
Cartrax, Peritrate

**Actions**
Relaxes muscle cells. Onset evident in 30–60 minutes.

**Uses**
Angina pectoris

**Contraindications**
Alcohol, children. *Use with caution:* Anemia, glaucoma, hypersensitivity to vasodilators, hyperthyroidism, intracranial pressure, MI

**Interactions**
Antihypertensives

**Dose**
*Adult*  Tablets: 10–40 mg qid; sustained-release: 80 mg bid

**Forms**
Sustained-release capsules, tablets

**Adverse Effects**
Blurred vision, dizziness, flushing, headache, nausea, orthostatic hypotension, vomiting

## Special Nursing Considerations and Patient Education

- Protect medication from heat and moisture.
- Be aware that
  - tolerance can develop.
- Teach patient to
  - not chew or crush sustained-release capsules.
  - take 30 minutes before or 1 hour after meals to decrease GI distress.
  - change position slowly to prevent orthostatic hypotension.
  - decrease smoking because it often potentiates angina pectoris attacks.
  - use caution in cold weather and during exercise when attacks may be worse.
  - identify stressors and ways to decrease them.
  - notify physician for blurred vision, skin rash.
  - notify physician if attacks increase.

# Pentazocine HCl

**Brand Name**
Talwin

**Actions**
Analgesic, sedative. Onset evident: IM, PO, SC 15–30 minutes; IV 2–3 minutes

**Uses**
Pain, sedation

**Contraindications**
*Meds* Alcohol, CNS depressants
*Other* Children under 12, head injury, increased intracranial pressure. *Use with caution:* Gallbladder disorders, hepatic or renal dysfunction, MI, narcotic dependence, prostatic hypertrophy, seizures, urethral stricture

**Interactions**
Anticholinergics, antidepressants, hypnotics, MAO inhibitors, meperidine, methadone, morphine, narcotics, sedatives, skeletal muscle relaxants, tranquilizers, tricyclic antidepressants

**Dose**
*Adult* PO: initial dose, 50 mg q3–4h; may be increased to 100 mg; *maximum* dose: 600 mg/day; IM/IV/SC: 30 mg q3–4h; *maximum* dose: 300 mg/day

**Forms**
Hydrochloride tablets, lactate injection

**Adverse Effects**
Blurred vision, diaphoresis, dizziness, drowsiness, dry mouth, nausea, vomiting

**Special Nursing Considerations
and Patient Education**
- Protect medication from direct light.
- Do not combine with soluble barbiturates in same syringe because precipitations will occur.
- Offer hard candy (regular or sugar-free) to relieve dry mouth.
- Be aware that
    - dependence is possible; when discontinued, decrease dosage gradually.
    - tolerance can develop.
    - IM and IV are preferred over SC when frequent injections are needed.
- Teach patient
    - to avoid alcohol and other depressants.
    - to be cautious when driving or involved in potentially hazardous tasks.

# Pentobarbital Sodium

**Brand Name**

Nembutal

**Actions**

Barbiturate, hypnotic, sedative. Onset evident in 15–20 minutes.

**Uses**

Insomnia, sedation

**Contraindications**

*Meds* Alcohol, CNS depressants

*Other* Hepatic or renal disease, porphyria, uncontrolled pain. *Use with caution:* Anemia (parenteral use), asthma, cardiovascular disease, diabetes, epilepsy, hyperkinesis, hypertension, hyperthyroidism (parenteral use), hypoadrenalism, hypotension, narrow-angle glaucoma, pulmonary or renal disease

**Interactions**

Chloramphenicol, corticosteroids, digitoxin, doxycycline, estradiol, griseofulvin, isoniazid, MAO inhibitors, oral anticoagulants or contraceptives, phenylbutazone, phenytoin, valproic acid

**Dose**

*Adult* PO: Hypnotic: 100–200 mg hs; sedative: 20–30 mg tid–qid; *maximum* dose: 120 mg/day

*Peds* PO: 6 mg/kg/day in 3 divided doses

**Forms**

Capsules, elixir, injection, long-acting tablets, suppositories

## Adverse Effects
Apnea, bronchospasm, hypotension, laryngospasm, respiratory depression

## Special Nursing Considerations and Patient Education
- Protect elixir from direct light.
- Administer hypnotic 15–30 minutes prior to hs.
- Administer IM dose slowly and deeply (no more than 5 cc at one site); observe for adverse effects for 30 minutes.
- Administer IV dose slowly; monitor vital signs q3–5min.
- Be aware that
  - medication is habit-forming; when discontinued, decrease dosage gradually.
- Teach patient
  - that medication may cause photosensitivity.
  - to be cautious when driving or involved in potentially hazardous tasks.

# Perphenazine

**Brand Name**
Trilafon

**Actions**
Antiemetic, antipsychotic

**Uses**
Acute or chronic schizophrenia; bipolar depression; involutional, senile, or toxic psychosis; nausea; vomiting

**Contraindications**
*Meds* Alcohol
*Other* Blood disorders, bone-marrow disorders, children under 12, hepatic impairment. *Use with caution:* Allergy to phenothiazines, cardiovascular disorders, epilepsy, glaucoma, Parkinson's disease, peptic ulcer, prostatic hypertrophy, respiratory disorder, urinary retention

**Interactions**
Amphetamines, antacids, anticonvulsants, antidiarrheals, antihistamines, atropine-like medications, CNS depressants, guanethidine, hypnotics, levodopa, MAO inhibitors, methyldopa, narcotics, reserpine, sedatives, tranquilizers, tricyclic antidepressants

**Dose**
*Adult* PO: 4–16 mg/day in 2–4 divided doses; IM: 5–10 mg q6h
*Peds* Over 12 yr: Same as adult

## Forms

Concentrate, injection, prolonged-action tablets, suppositories, syrup, tablets

## Adverse Effects

Blurred vision, constipation, dermatitis, dizziness, dry mouth, extrapyramidal symptoms, orthostatic hypotension, sedation, syncope

## Special Nursing Considerations and Patient Education

- Protect liquid forms from direct light.
- Do not crush prolonged-action tablets.
- Dilute concentrate; avoid using apple or grape juice, coffee, cola, tea.
- Administer IM dose slowly and deeply; have patient remain recumbent for ½ hour; massage injection site.
- Avoid administering IV dose in undiluted form; administer slowly as directed.
- When discontinued, decrease dosage gradually.
- Monitor for fine vermicular tongue movements (may indicate early tardive dyskinesia).
- Offer hard candy (regular or sugar-free) to relieve dry mouth.
- Teach patient
  - that medication may cause photosensitivity.
  - to be cautious when driving or involved in potentially hazardous tasks.

# Phenazopyridine HCl/Sulfisoxazole

**Brand Name**
Azo Gantrisin

**Actions**
Analgesic, sulfonamide; hinders synthesis of folic acid by susceptible bacteria

**Uses**
Painful infections of urinary tract

**Contraindications**
Children under 12, glomerulonephritis, hypersensitivity to sulfa drugs, severe hepatitis, uremia. *Use with caution:* Allergies, bronchial asthma, hepatic or renal impairment

**Interactions**
Phenylbutazone, phenytoin, salicylates, tolbutamide, warfarin

**Dose**
*Adult* Initial dose: 4–6 tablets; then 2 tablets qid, up to 3/day

**Forms**
Tablets

**Adverse Effects**
Anorexia, depression, diarrhea, hallucinations, headache, hepatitis, nausea, tinnitus, vertigo, vomiting

**Special Nursing Considerations
and Patient Education**
- Monitor acidity of patient's urine; may require a
  urinary alkalizer.
- Teach patient
  - that medication will discolor urine orange or red.
  - to keep well hydrated.
  - that medication may cause photosensitivity.

# Phenelzine Sulfate

**Brand Name**
Nardil

**Actions**
MAO inhibitor. Onset evident in 1–2 weeks.

**Uses**
Endogenous or reactive depression, involutional melancholia

**Contraindications**

*Meds* Alcohol, amphetamines, CNS depressants, dopamine, epinephrine, levodopa, methyldopa, norepinephrine, tryptophan, tyramine

*Other* Arteriosclerosis, atonic colitis, cardiovascular disease, cerebrovascular disease, children under 16, elderly over 60, epilepsy, hepatic impairment, hypernatremia, hypertension, hyperthyroidism, paranoid schizophrenia, pheochromocytoma. *Use with caution:* Convulsive disorders, glaucoma

**Interactions**
Antihypertensives, barbiturates, general anesthesia, oral hypoglycemic agents, reserpine, tricyclic antidepressants

**Dose**

*Adult* 15 mg tid; *maximum* dose: 75 mg/day; *maintenance* dose: 15 mg qd-qod

**Forms**
Tablets

**Adverse Effects**
Constipation, dizziness, drowsiness, dry mouth, GI disturbances, insomnia, orthostatic hypotension, tremors

## Special Nursing Considerations and Patient Education

- Protect medication from light and heat.
- Use caution when administering to a patient with suicidal potential; ensure patient swallows dose.
- When discontinued, decrease dosage gradually.
- Monitor blood pressure, I&O, weight; for diabetic patients monitor for evidence of hypoglycemia.
- Offer hard candy (regular or sugar-free) to relieve dry mouth.
- Give diet that does not contain foods high in tryptophan and tyramine (see Appendix F).
- Teach patient to
  - change position slowly to decrease hypotension.
  - limit caffeine intake.
  - continue diet restrictions for 2 weeks after medication is discontinued.

# Phenobarbital, Phenobarbital Sodium

## Brand Name
Phenobarbital

## Actions
Hypnotic, sedative; reduces nerve impulses to cerebral cortex through action on brainstem reticular formation. Onset evident in 1 hour.

## Uses
Insomnia, seizures (focal, grand mal, status epilepticus)

## Contraindications
*Meds* Alcohol, CNS depressants

*Other* Hepatic dysfunction, latent porphyria. *Use with caution:* Anemia; asthma; borderline hypoadrenalism; cardiac, renal, or hepatic impairment; diabetes; epilepsy; hyperkinesis; hypertension or hyperthyroidism (parenteral use)

## Interactions
Anticoagulants, chloramphenicol, corticosteroids, digitoxin, doxycycline, estradiol, griseofulvin, isoniazid, MAO inhibitors, oral contraceptives, phenylbutazone, phenytoin, valproic acid

## Dose
*Adult* PO: Sedative: 16–32 mg; hypnotic: 100 mg hs

*Peds* PO: Sedative: 6 mg/kg/day in 3 divided doses; hypnotic: 3–6 mg/kg hs

## Forms
Elixir, prolonged-action capsules, injection, tablets

## Adverse Effects

Apnea, bradycardia, confusion, depression, diarrhea, dizziness, excitement, nausea, somnolence, vomiting

## Special Nursing Considerations and Patient Education

- Protect liquid forms from light.
- Do not crush prolonged-action capsules.
- Administer IM deeply into muscle.
- When IV form used, monitor patient constantly for rapid change in condition.
- Use caution when administering to a patient with suicidal potential; ensure patient swallows dose.
- Be aware that
  - medication can be habit-forming; when discontinued, decrease dosage gradually.
  - cross tolerance to barbiturates is possible.
- Teach patient
  - that medication may cause photosensitivity.
  - to notify physician of fever, hemorrhage, jaundice, rash, sore throat.
  - to be cautious when driving or involved in potentially hazardous tasks.

# Phenylbutazone

**Brand Name**
Azolid, Butazolidin

**Actions**
Analgesic, anti-inflammatory, antipyretic. Onset evident in 30-60 minutes.

**Uses**
Ankylosing spondylitis, bursitis, gout, osteo-arthritis, peritendinitis, psoriasis, rheumatoid arthritis, superficial thrombophlebitis

**Contraindications**
*Meds* Alcohol, oral anticoagulants
*Other* Allergy to any medication; cardiac, hepatic, renal or thyroid dysfunction; children under 14; edema; history of blood dyscrasias, bone-marrow disease, cardiac decompensation, peptic ulcer or stomach ulceration; hypertension; persistent dyspepsia; polymyalgia rheumatica; senility; temporal arteritis. *Use with caution:* Glaucoma

**Interactions**
Acetohexamide, antidiabetics, antihistamines, anti-inflammatories, aspirin, barbiturates, cholestyramine, digitalis, indomethacin, insulin, oral contraceptives, phenytoin, steroids, sulfonamides, sulfonylureas, tricyclic antidepressants

**Dose**
*Adult* 200-400 mg/day in 3-4 divided doses; *maximum* dose: 400 mg/day

**Forms**
Capsules, enteric-coated tablets

## Adverse Effects

Abdominal discomfort, diarrhea, dizziness, dyspepsia, edema, hearing impairment, hematuria, hypertension, nausea, peptic ulcer, proteinuria, rash

## Special Nursing Considerations and Patient Education

- Monitor I&O, weight.
- Teach patient
  - to take medication at meals or with milk to decrease GI irritation.
  - to notify physician after 7 days if there is no favorable response.
  - that medication may cause photosensitivity.
  - to be cautious when driving or involved in potentially hazardous tasks.
  - to notify physician for black stools, blurred vision, edema, fever, oral lesions, salivary gland enlargement, sore throat, weight gain.

# Phenytoin, Phenytoin Sodium

## Brand Name
Dilantin, Dilantin Infantab, Dilantin 30 Pediatric

## Actions
Anticonvulsant; promotes sodium efflux from neurons, which then hinders motor cortex seizure activity. Onset evident: PO 8 hours; IV 5 minutes.

## Uses
Digitalis-induced dysrhythmias, grand mal or psychomotor seizures, migraine or trigeminal neuralgia pain

## Contraindications
*Meds* Alcohol
*Other* Adams-Stokes syndrome, atrioventricular block, hepatic disease, sinoatrial block, sinus bradycardia

## Interactions
Antidepressants, antihistamines, aspirin, barbiturates, chloramphenicol, chlordiazepoxide, CNS depressants, corticosteroids, cortisone, cycloserine, digitalis, disulfiram, doxycycline, estrogens, folic acid antagonists, glutethemide, griseofulvin, hypnotics, hypoglycemics, isoniazid, levodopa, lidocaine, methotrexate, methylphenidate, oral anticoagulants or contraceptives, oxyphenbutazone, para-aminosalicylic acid, phenothiazines, phenylbutazone, propranolol, quinidine, sedatives, sulfa medications, sympathomimetics, tranquilizers, tubocurarine, valproic acid

## Dose

*Adult* PO: initial dose, 100 mg tid; *maintenance* dose: 300–600 mg/day

*Peds* PO: initial dose, 5 mg/kg/day in 2–3 divided doses; *maximum* dose: 300 mg/day; *maintenance* dose: 4–8 mg/kg/day

## Forms

Capsules, injection, suspension, tablets

## Adverse Effects

Ataxia, confusion, constipation, dizziness, extrapyramidal symptoms, gingival hyperplasia, hallucinations, headache, insomnia, nausea, nervousness, nystagmus, tremors, vomiting

## Special Nursing Considerations and Patient Education

- Administer exactly as directed; do not exceed 50 mg/minute; follow injection with saline to avoid irritation of vein.
- Take pulse prior to administration of IV dose and compare with patient's guidelines.
- Administer IM dose deep into large muscle.
- Administer oral dose with a ½ glass of water immediately before or after meals to decrease GI distress.
- Monitor blood pressure, pulse, respiration; for diabetic patients, monitor for signs of hyperglycemia (see Appendix B).
- When discontinued, decrease dosage gradually.

*(continued)*

# Phenytoin, Phenytoin Sodium (continued)

- Be aware that
  - there is a small margin between therapeutic and toxic levels.
- Teach patient
  - that medication may turn urine brown, pink, or red.
  - to avoid alcohol.
  - to notify physician if becomes ill, and for fever, rash, sore throat.
  - to be cautious when driving or involved in potentially hazardous tasks.
  - to maintain proper oral hygiene because of possible gingival hyperplasia.
- Teach patient and family
  - regarding possibility of seizures

# NOTES

# Piperacetazine

**Brand Name**
Quide

**Actions**
Antipsychotic, tranquilizer

**Uses**
Acute or chronic schizophrenia, psychotic
disorders

**Contraindications**
*Meds* Alcohol
*Other* Blood dyscrasias, children under 12, coma,
depression, hepatic disease. *Use with caution:*
Epilepsy

**Interactions**
Amphetamines, antacids, anticonvulsants,
antidiarrheals, antihistamines, atropine-like
medications, CNS depressants, guanethidine,
hypnotics, levodopa, MAO inhibitors, methyldopa,
narcotics, reserpine, sedatives, tranquilizers,
tricyclic antidepressants

**Dose**
*Adult* Individualized, initial dose: 10 mg bid–qid;
gradually increase over 3–5 days; *maximum*
dose: 160 mg/day
*Peds* Over 12 yr: same as adults

**Forms**
Tablets

**Adverse Effects**
Constipation, decreased libido, dermatitis,
dizziness, drowsiness, extrapyramidal symptoms,
orthostatic hypotension, syncope

**Special Nursing Considerations
and Patient Education**
- Protect medication from light.
- Monitor for fine vermicular tongue movements (may indicate early tardive dyskinesia).
- Teach patient
  - that medication may cause photosensitivity.
  - to change position slowly to decrease hypotension.
  - to be cautious when driving or involved in potentially hazardous tasks.

# Polymixin B Sulfate

**Brand Name**
Aerosporin

**Actions**
Antibiotic; disrupts cell membrane in susceptible microorganisms

**Uses**
Infections (susceptible microorganisms that are resistant to less toxic antibiotics)

**Contraindications**
*Meds* Amikacin, colistimethate, colistin, gentamicin, kanamycin, nephrotoxics, streptomycin, tobramycin, viomycin
*Other* Nitrogen retention, renal impairment

**Interactions**
Anesthetics, neuromuscular blocking agents, skeletal muscle relaxants

**Dose**
*Adult* IM: 25,000–30,000 U/kg/day in divided doses; IV: 15,000–25,000 U/kg/day
*Peds* Same as adult

**Forms**
Injection, ophthalmic solution, otic drops, topical powder

**Adverse Effects**
Blurred vision, dizziness, drug fever, hematuria, irritability, nausea, neurologic disturbances, peripheral paresthesia, transient albuminuria, vomiting

**Special Nursing Considerations
and Patient Education**
- Store parenteral forms in refrigerator.
- Administer exactly per manufacturer's directions.
- Evaluate renal function prior to administration.
- Monitor patient's temperature.
- Be aware that
  - IM route is usually not recommended; if used, rotate sites.
- Teach patient to
  - notify physician of blurred vision, dizziness, numbness, pruritus, speech slurring, tingling, urinary problems.

# Prednisone

**Brand Name**
Deltasone, Sterapred

**Actions**
Anti-inflammatory; inhibits immune response

**Uses**
Allergies; collagen, dermatologic, respiratory, or rheumatic diseases; hematologic or ophthalmologic disorders; palliative measure for leukemia; primary or secondary adrenocortical insufficiency

**Contraindications**
Active tuberculosis, eye infections due to herpes simplex virus, infections uncontrolled by antibiotics, psychosis, systemic fungal infection. *Use with caution:* Cardiac disorder, cirrhosis, diabetes, emotional instability, fresh intestinal anastomosis, glaucoma, hepatic dysfunction, herpes simplex (ocular), history of tuberculosis, hypertension, hypothyroidism, myasthenia gravis, osteoporosis, peptic ulcer, pyrogenic infections, renal insufficiency, ulcerative colitis

**Interactions**
Aspirin, ephedrine, insulin, oral anticoagulants or hypoglycemic agents, phenobarbital, phenytoin, potassium-depleting diuretics, rifampin

**Dose**
*Adult*  Initial dose: 30–60 mg/day in 2–4 divided doses; after 2–7 days, *decrease* gradually by 5–10 mg to a *maintenance* dose of 5–20 mg/day

*Peds*  Initial dose: 2 mg/kg/day in 4 divided doses; decrease *gradually* over 2–3 weeks to a *maintenance* dose of 1.5 mg/kg/day

**Forms**
　Tablets

**Adverse Effects**
　Abdominal distention, blurred vision, electrolyte
　disturbance, hypotension, increased intracranial
　pressure, mood changes, nausea, osteoporosis,
　petechiae, purpura, vomiting

**Special Nursing Considerations
and Patient Education**
- Protect medication from air and direct light.
- Monitor weight, potassium levels periodically.
- Be aware that
  - dependence is possible; when discontinued,
    decrease dosage gradually.
- Teach patient to
  - ingest a diet high in potassium and protein but
    low in salt.
  - take medications after meals and at hs.
  - carry some type of Medic Alert card or bracelet.
  - avoid stress as much as possible.
  - notify physician of abdominal pain, confusion,
    hypotension, illness.

# Primidone

**Brand Name**
Mysoline

**Actions**
Anticonvulsant; changes seizure patterns;
increases seizure threshold through action on CNS

**Uses**
Grand mal, myoclonic, or psychomotor seizures

**Contraindications**
*Meds* Alcohol
*Other* Hypersensitivity to phenobarbital, porphyria,
purpura. *Use with caution:* History of hepatic
or renal disease, hyperkinesia, lupus
erythematosus, respiratory disease

**Interactions**
Barbiturates, isoniazid, phenytoin

**Dose**
*Adult* Individualized; 250 mg/day; increase weekly by
250 mg; *maximum* dose: 500 mg qid
*Peds* Individualized; under 8 yr: ½ of adult dose;
over 8 yr: Same as adult

**Forms**
Suspension, tablets

**Adverse Effects**
Alopecia, ataxia, diplopia, drowsiness, impotence,
irritability, mood changes, nausea, nystagmus,
vertigo, vomiting

### Special Nursing Considerations
### and Patient Education
- Protect liquid forms from light.
- When discontinued, decrease dosage gradually.
- Document seizure activity fully.
- Be aware that
  - transfer from other anticonvulsants should require a 2-month transition period.
- Teach patient to
  - carry some type of Medic Alert card or bracelet.
  - be cautious when driving or involved in potentially hazardous tasks.
  - notify physician if becomes ill or for rash.

# Procainamide HCl

**Brand Name**
Pronestyl

**Actions**
Antidysrhythmic; decreases cardiac automaticity, conductivity, and excitability. Onset evident: PO 30 minutes; IV immediately.

**Uses**
Digitalis intoxication, dysrhythmias (atrial fibrillation, paroxysmal atrial tachycardia, premature ventricular contractions, ventricular tachycardia)

**Contraindications**
Allergies, blood dyscrasias, cardiac damage, complete atrioventricular heart block, myasthenia gravis, 2nd or 3rd degree atrioventricular block. *Use with caution:* Allergy to chemically related medications; asthma; hepatic or renal dysfunction; lupus erythematosus

**Interactions**
Ammonium chloride, cholinergics, digitalis, isoniazid, lidocaine, skeletal muscle relaxants, sodium bicarbonate

**Dose**
*Adult* PO: Initial dose: 1 gm; *maintenance* dose: 50 mg/kg/day q3h
*Peds* PO: 50 mg/kg in 4–6 divided doses

**Forms**
Capsules, injection, tablets

**Adverse Effects**

Anorexia, depression, diarrhea, hallucinations, lupus erythematosis syndrome, nausea, psychosis, urticaria, vomiting

**Special Nursing Considerations and Patient Education**

- Discard solutions if darker than light amber or otherwise discolored.
- Protect vials from light and temperature changes.
- Discontinue if diastolic blood pressure is below 15 mm Hg.
- Monitor urinary output, vital signs; with IV, constantly monitor blood pressure, EKG.
- Be aware that
  - plasma levels should be 4–8 mcg/ml.
  - that medication is cumulative.
- Teach patient
  - to take with food to decrease GI upset.
  - to decrease intake of caffeine and iced drinks because of their stimulant effect.
  - that medication may cause a bitter taste in mouth.
  - to carry some type of Medic Alert card or bracelet.
  - to be cautious when driving or involved in potentially hazardous tasks.
  - to notify physician of fever, hemorrhage, rash, respiratory tract infection, sore throat.

# Promazine HCl

**Brand Name**
Sparine

**Actions**
Sedative, tranquilizer. Onset evident in 1–2 hours.

**Uses**
Alcohol-induced hallucinations, delirium tremens, drug withdrawal, nausea, psychosis, vomiting

**Contraindications**
*Meds* Alcohol
*Other* Blood disorders, bone-marrow disorders, children under 12. *Use with caution:* Cardiac disease, epilepsy, hepatic or respiratory disease, parkinsonism, peptic ulcer, prostatic hypertrophy

**Interactions**
Amphetamines, antacids, anticonvulsants, antidiarrheals, antihistamines, atropine-like medications, CNS depressants, guanethidine, hypnotics, levodopa, MAO inhibitors, methyldopa, narcotics, reserpine, sedatives, tranquilizers, tricyclic antidepressants

**Dose**
*Adult* PO: 10–200 mg q4–6h; *maximum* dose: 1,000 mg/day
*Peds* PO: Over 12 yr: 10–25 mg q4–6h

**Forms**
Concentrate, injection, syrup, tablets

## Adverse Effects

Constipation, drowsiness, extrapyramidal symptoms, leukopenia, orthostatic hypotension, sedation, syncope

## Special Nursing Considerations and Patient Education

- Protect medication from direct light.
- Administer injections slowly; have patient lie down for 30 minutes after administration.
- Dilute concentrate with carbonated drinks or fruit juices.
- When discontinued, decrease dosage gradually.
- Monitor for fine vermicular tongue movements (may indicate early tardive dyskinesia).
- Teach patient
  - to change position slowly to decrease hypotension.
  - that medication may cause photosensitivity.
  - that urine may turn pink or purple.
  - to be cautious when driving or involved in potentially hazardous tasks.
  - to use caution in hot weather because of potential orthostatic hypotension.

# Promethazine HCl

**Brand Name**
Phenergan, Remsed

**Actions**
Histamine antagonist. Onset evident: PO 1–2 hours.

**Uses**
Adjunct for anaphylactic reaction or pain; allergic reactions; apprehension; motion sickness; obstetrics; pre- and postoperatively

**Contraindications**
*Meds* Alcohol
*Other* Blood or bone-marrow disorders, narrow-angle glaucoma, neonates. *Use with caution:* Allergy to phenothiazines, children with flu symptoms, peptic ulcer, prostatic hypertrophy

**Interactions**
Amphetamines, antacids, anticonvulsants, antidiarrheals, antihistamines, atropine-like medications, CNS depressants, guanethidine, hypnotics, levodopa, MAO inhibitors, methyldopa, narcotics, reserpine, sedatives, tranquilizers, tricyclic antidepressants

**Dose**
*Adult* Individualized; PO: 12.5–150 mg qd in divided doses
*Peds* Individualized; PO: 0.25–0.5 mg/kg/day

**Forms**
Injection, suppositories, syrup, tablets

**Adverse Effects**
Blurred vision, confusion, dizziness, drowsiness, dry mouth, hypotension, sedation

## Special Nursing Considerations and Patient Education

- Protect medication from light.
- Monitor respirations for patient with respiratory problems.
- For motion sickness, administer initial dose ½–1 hour prior to travel.
- Offer hard candy (regular or sugar-free) to relieve dry mouth.
- Administer with food to decrease irritation.
- Be aware that
  - IM is preferred parenteral route; administer into deep muscle.
  - IV concentration should be less than 25 mg/cc; rate should be no more than 25 mg/minute.
- Teach patient
  - that medication may color urine brown, pink, or red.
  - to be cautious when driving or involved in potentially hazardous tasks.
  - to not take nonprescription medications without notifying physician.
  - to notify physician for ecchymosis, fever, rash, skin discoloration, sore throat, tremors, vision impairment.

# Propoxyphene HCl

**Brand Name**
Darvon

**Actions**
Analgesic; increases pain threshold. Onset evident in 1–2 hours.

**Uses**
Pain

**Contraindications**
Alcohol, children, CNS depressants. *Use with caution:* Hepatic or renal disease

**Interactions**
Alcohol, carbamazepine, CNS depressants, oral anticoagulants, orphenadrine

**Dose**
*Adult* 65 mg qid

**Forms**
Capsules

**Adverse Effects**
Constipation, dizziness, drowsiness, headache, nausea, sedation, vomiting

## Special Nursing Considerations and Patient Education

- Be aware that
  - dependence is possible; when discontinued, decrease dosage gradually.
  - tolerance can develop.
- Teach patient to
  - decrease smoking as it affects drug metabolism.
  - be cautious when driving or involved in potentially hazardous tasks.

# Propranolol

**Brand Name**
Inderal

**Actions**
Antianginal, antidysrhythmic, antihypertensive, beta-adrenergic blocking agent. Onset evident: PO 30 minutes–1 hour; IV 3–5 minutes.

**Uses**
Adjunct for pheochromocytoma, angina pectoris, cardiac dysrhythmias, hypertension, hypertrophic subaortic stenosis, migraine

**Contraindications**
*Meds* Adrenergic-augmenting psychotropics, alcohol, furazolidone, general anesthetics, MAO inhibitors

*Other* Atrioventricular heart block, bronchial asthma, children, congestive heart failure, hypotension, rhinitis, right ventricular failure, sinus bradycardia. *Use with caution:* Bradycardia, bronchospasm (nonallergic), cardiovascular disease, diabetes, emphysema, hay fever, hepatic or renal impairment, hyperthyroid, hypoglycemia, Reynaud's syndrome, Wolff-Parkinson-White syndrome

**Interactions**
Aminophylline, anti-inflammatories, cimetidine, digitalis, dobutamine, dopamine, guanethidine, isoproterenol, MAO inhibitors, norepinephrine, oral antidiabetics, phenytoin, reserpine

**Dose**
*Adult* PO: Initial dose: 10–20 mg tid–qid; *maintenance* dose: 160–640 mg/day

**Forms**

Injection, tablets

**Adverse Effects**

Bradycardia, congestive heart failure, constipation, depression, diarrhea, hallucinations, hypoglycemia, lethargy, nausea, orthostatic hypotension, respiratory distress, vomiting

**Special Nursing Considerations and Patient Education**

- Protect medication from light.
- Take apical/radial pulse prior to administration and compare with patient's guidelines.
- Administer IV dose slowly.
- Give oral medication before meals and at hs.
- Monitor blood pressure, I&O, neurologic status, renal function, vital signs, weight.
- For IV route, withhold other medications for 4 hours after dose; monitor EKG.
- Have atropine available in case of hypotension.
- When discontinued, decrease dosage gradually.
- Teach patient to
  - decrease caffeine and smoking because of their impact on blood pressure.
  - be cautious when driving or involved in potentially hazardous tasks.
  - be cautious in cold weather and during strenuous exercise because of their impact on circulation.
  - notify physician for edema, respiratory distress, or if becomes ill.

# Protriptyline HCl

**Brand Name**
Vivactil

**Actions**
Tricyclic antidepressant. Onset evident in 1–2 weeks.

**Uses**
Endogenous or exogenous depression

**Contraindications**
*Meds* Alcohol, MAO inhibitors
*Other* Children, closed-angle glaucoma, prostatic hypertrophy, pyloric stenosis, recent MI, renal disease, urinary retention. *Use with caution:* Asthma, cardiovascular or GI disorders, diabetes, epilepsy, glaucoma, hepatic or thryoid function impairment

**Interactions**
Adrenergics, anticholinergics, anticonvulsants, antihistamines, antihypertensives, atropine-like medications, clonidine, CNS depressants, estrogens, ethchlorvynol, guanethidine, hypnotics, levodopa, narcotics, procainamide, quinidine, sedatives, sympathomimetics, thyroid preparations, tranquilizers

**Dose**
*Adult* Individualized; 5–10 mg tid–qid; *maximum* dose: 60 mg/day

**Forms**
Tablets

## Adverse Effects

Anorexia, dizziness, drowsiness, dry mouth, extrapyramidal symptoms, headache, insomnia, nausea, orthostatic hypotension, paresthesia, tremors, vomiting, weakness

## Special Nursing Considerations and Patient Education

- When administering to patients with insomnia, administer last daily dose prior to midafternoon.
- When increasing dosage, increase morning dose to reduce sleep disruption.
- Use caution when administering to a patient with suicidal potential; ensure patient swallows dose.
- Monitor vital signs until dosage is stabilized.
- Offer hard candy (regular or sugar-free) to relieve dry mouth.
- When discontinued, decrease dosage gradually.
- Teach patient
  - that medication may cause photosensitivity.
  - to change position slowly to prevent orthostatic hypotension.
  - to be cautious when driving or involved in potentially hazardous tasks.

# Pseudoephedrine HCl/
# Triprolidine HCl

**Brand Name**
Actifed

**Actions**
Antihistamine, decongestant

**Uses**
Allergic or vasomotor rhinitis, upper respiratory difficulties

**Contraindications**
Hypersensitivity. *Use with caution:* Hypertension

**Interactions**
Ephedrine, stimulants

**Dose**
*Adult* 10 cc or 1 tablet tid-qid
*Peds* 1.25-5 cc tid-qid

**Forms**
Syrup, tablets

**Adverse Effects**
Drowsiness, stimulation

**Special Nursing Considerations
and Patient Education**
- Protect medication from direct light.
- Teach patient
  - to be cautious when driving or involved in potentially hazardous tasks.

# Quinidine

## Brand Name
Cin-Quin, Quinora

## Actions
Antidysrhythmic; delays electrical impulse transmission; decreases pacemaker activity. Onset evident in 1–3 hours.

## Uses
Atrial flutter, nocturnal cramps, paroxysmal atrial fibrillation, paroxysmal atrial or ventricular tachycardia, premature atrial or ventricular contractions

## Contraindications
Atrioventricular block, digitalis intoxication, dysrhythmia, history of thrombocytopenic purpura, intraventricular conduction defects. *Use with caution:* Acute infections, asthma, bradycardia, cardiac enlargement, chronic valvular disease, congestive heart failure, coronary occlusion, hepatic or renal insufficiency, history of angina pectoris or hyperthyroidism, hypokalemia, incomplete AV block, MI, myasthenia gravis, psoriasis, subacute endocarditis

## Interactions
Acetazolamide, antacids, anticholinergics, digoxin, neuromuscular-blocking agents, oral anti-coagulants, phenobarbital, phenytoin, rifampin, sodium bicarbonate, thiazide diuretics, verapamil, warfarin

## Dose
*Adult*  Individualized; PO: 1–2 sustained-release tablets q8–12h; IM: initial dose, 600 mg, then 400 mg q2h

*Peds*  PO: Test dose of 2 mg/kg; *therapeutic* dose: 6
mg/kg/5x/day

## Forms

Gluconate or sulfate injection, sulfate tablets,
sustained-release tablets containing gluconate or
sulfate

## Adverse Effects

Bradycardia, cinchonism, confusion, hypotension,
nausea, syncope, vomiting

## Special Nursing Considerations
## and Patient Education

- Protect medication from heat and light.
- Take blood pressure, apical pulse rate and rhythm,
  radial pulse (one minute) prior to administration
  and compare with patient's guidelines.
- Monitor I&O, serum concentration of medication.
- Administer one hour before or two hours after
  meals to maximize absorption.
- Give with food (but not with a full meal) to
  decrease GI upset.
- Be aware that
  - sustained-release tablets should be taken only
    for maintenance and prophylaxis.
- Teach patient
  - to decrease caffeine intake and smoking
    because of their stimulant effect.
  - to carry a Medic Alert card or bracelet.
  - to change position slowly to decrease
    hypotension.
  - may cause a bitter taste in mouth.
  - to notify physician of fever, hemorrhage, rash,
    tinnitus, visual disturbances.

# Reserpine

**Brand Name**
Serpasil

**Actions**
Antihypertensive, tranquilizer; lessens catecholamine depletion from peripheral tissues

**Uses**
Hypertension, psychiatric conditions

**Contraindications**
*Meds* Alcohol, CNS depressants
*Other* Active peptic ulcer, depression, ECT, ulcerative colitis. *Use with caution:* Gallstones; GI disorders; history of depression or peptic ulcer; renal insufficiency

**Interactions**
Anticonvulsants, antihistamines, digitalis, hypnotics, MAO inhibitors, narcotics, oral anticoagulants, phenothiazines, propranolol, quinidine, sedatives, tranquilizers

**Dose**
*Adult* PO: Initial dose: 0.5 mg/day x 1–2 weeks; *maintenance* dose: 0.1–0.25 mg/day
*Peds* PO: 0.07 mg/kg/day in 2 divided doses

**Forms**
Capsules, injection, tablets

**Adverse Effects**
Bradycardia, depression, diarrhea, drowsiness, lethargy, nasal congestion, nausea, weight gain

## Special Nursing Considerations
## and Patient Education

- Protect medication from direct light.
- Check blood pressure prior to administration.
- Administer after meals, or with food/milk, to decrease GI upset.
- Monitor blood pressure, I&O, neurologic status, weight.
- Teach patient to
  - be cautious when driving or involved in potentially hazardous tasks.
  - follow suggested diet.
  - notify physician at first evidence of depression (e.g., early morning insomnia, feeling down, sad affect), or mood changes.

# Scopolamine Hydrobromide

## Actions
Anticholinergic, antimuscarinic, cycloplegic, mydriatic, parasympatholytic, salivary inhibitor; competes with acetylcholine for muscarinic receptors

## Uses
Motion sickness, obstetrics, parkinsonism, surgery

## Contraindications
Adhesions of iris and lens, asthma, hepatic or renal impairment, hiatal hernia, reflux esophagitis, intestinal atony, myasthenia gravis, narrow-angle glaucoma, obstructive diseases of GI or urinary tract, toxemias, ulcerative colitis. *Use with caution:* Chronic lung disease

## Interactions
Antihistamines, cholinergics, digitalis, levodopa, MAO inhibitors, narcotics, phenothiazines, quinidine, tricyclic antidepressants

## Dose
*Adult* PO: 0.5–1 mg;.IM/IV/SC: 0.3–0.6 mg
*Peds* PO: SC: 0.006 mg/kg

## Forms
Injection, tablets

## Adverse Effects
Blurred vision, disorientation, dizziness, dry mouth, respiratory depression

**Special Nursing Considerations
and Patient Education**
- Protect medication from light.
- Be aware that tolerance can develop.
- Do not administer alone for pain; give with an analgesic.
- Monitor vital signs.
- Offer hard candy (regular or sugar-free) to relieve dry mouth.
- Teach patient
  - to be cautious when driving or involved in potentially hazardous tasks.
  - to increase fluid intake and bulk in diet to decrease constipation.

# Secobarbital Sodium

**Brand Name**
Seconal

**Actions**
Hypnotic, sedative; lessens available norepinephrine. Onset evident in 30 minutes.

**Uses**
Acute convulsive disorders, insomnia, pre-operative

**Contraindications**
Alcohol. *Use with caution:* Anemia, cardiac disease, diabetes, epilepsy, hyperkinesis, hypertension, hyperthyroid, hypoadrenalism, pain, renal or respiratory disease

**Interactions**
Anticonvulsants; antidepressants; antihistamines; cortisone, digitalis; digitoxin, griseofulvin; hypnotics; isoniazid, MAO inhibitors; narcotics; oral anticoagulants, contraceptives, or antidiabetics; phenylbutazone; phenytoin; sedatives; tranquilizers

**Dose**
*Adult*  Hypnotic: 100–200 mg PO, IM; sedative: 30–50 mg tid PO
*Peds*  Hypnotic: 3–5 mg/kg PO; sedative: 6 mg/kg/day PO in 3 divided doses

**Forms**
Capsules, elixir, injection, suppositories, tablets

**Adverse Effects**
Bradycardia, dizziness, drowsiness, excitement, hypoventilation, nausea, vomiting

## Special Nursing Considerations
## and Patient Education
- Protect elixir from light.
- Store suppositories in refrigerator.
- Administer IM into deep muscle mass.
- Monitor blood pressure, pulse, respirations: IM for 20-30 minutes; IV constantly, with respirations every 3-5 minutes.
- Be aware that
  - parenteral solutions must be clear.
  - dependence is possible; when discontinued, decrease dosage gradually.
- Teach patient
  - that medication may cause photosensitivity.
  - to be cautious when driving or involved in potentially hazardous tasks.

# Spironolactone

**Brand Name**
  Aldactone

**Actions**
  Antihypertensive, potassium-sparing diuretic;
  blocks selected effects of aldosterone

**Uses**
  Edema, adrenal hyperplasia or adenomas,
  essential hypertension, hypokalemia

**Contraindications**
*Meds*  Potassium supplements
*Other*  Anuria, hyperkalemia, renal disorders. *Use
     with caution:* Hepatic disease, renal
     impairment

**Interactions**
  Anticoagulants, antihypertensives, digitalis
  glycosides, diuretics, ganglionic blocking agents,
  norepinephrine, triamterene

**Dose**
*Adult*  25–200 mg/day in divided doses
*Peds*  1.5–3.3 mg/kg/day in 4 divided doses

**Forms**
  Tablets

**Adverse Effects**
  Anorexia, ataxia, confusion, cramping, drowsiness,
  headache, hyperkalemia, hyponatremia,
  impotence, lethargy, menstrual irregularity, nausea

## Special Nursing Considerations
## and Patient Education

- Protect medication from direct light.
- Monitor blood pressure, electrolytes, I&O, weight.
- Observe patient for signs and symptoms of hyperkalemia or hyponatremia (see Appendix B).
- Discontinue for electrolyte imbalance.
- Teach patient
  - to avoid potassium-rich foods and salt substitutes (see Appendix F).
  - to be cautious when driving or involved in potentially hazardous tasks.
  - that full effect of medication does not occur for several days.
  - notify physician of gynecomastia, hirsutism, hyperkalemia, hyponatremia, impotence, menstrual irregularity.

# Streptomycin Sulfate

## Actions
Antibacterial, antibiotic, anti-infective, antitubercular; inhibits synthesis of ribosomal protein in susceptible microorganisms

## Uses
Bubonic plague, cholera, endocarditis (alpha-, bacterial, enterococcal, nonhemolytic streptococcal), tuberculosis, tularemia

## Contraindications
Contact or exfoliative dermatitis, myasthenia gravis. *Use with caution:* Eighth cranial nerve impairment, parkinsonism, renal impairment

## Interactions
Aminoglycosides, anesthetics, cephaloridine, cephalothin sodium, cisplatin, colistin, ethacrynic acid, furosemide, neuromuscular blocking agents, penicillins, polymixin B, vancomycin

## Dose
*Adult* Individualized; 1–4 gm in divided doses
*Peds* Individualized; 10–30 mg/kg/day in divided doses

## Forms
Injection

## Adverse Effects
Headache, hearing impairment, nephrotoxicity, paresthesias, respiratory depression

## Special Nursing Considerations
## and Patient Education
- Protect medication from direct light.
- Weigh patient prior to start of treatment to obtain a baseline weight.
- Protect hands while preparing dose.
- Do not administer solutions stronger than 500 mg/cc.
- Administer IM into deep muscle mass.
- Rotate injection sites.
- Monitor creatinine clearance; eighth cranial nerve function; hearing; I&O; presence of blood cells, casts in urine.
- Be aware that
  - medication is utilized for tuberculosis only in combination with other medications.
- Teach patient to
  - maintain good hydration (drink at least 10–12 glasses of fluid per day).
  - notify physician of hearing impairment.

# Sulfadiazine

**Brand Name**
Microdiazine, Microsulfon

**Actions**
Antiprotozoal, antitrypanosomal

**Uses**
Dysentery, infection of urinary tract, meningitis, rheumatic fever prophylaxis

**Contraindications**
Glomerulonephritis, hepatic or renal failure, hypersensitivity to sulfa drugs

**Interactions**
Chlorpropamide, methotrexate, phenylbutazone, phenytoin, probenecid, salicylates, tolbutamide, warfarin

**Dose**
*Adult* 2–4 gm/day
*Peds* 75–150 mg/kg/day in 4–6 divided doses

**Forms**
Tablets

**Adverse Effects**
Crystalluria, drowsiness, headache, hematuria, nausea, pruritus, urticaria, vomiting

## Special Nursing Considerations
## and Patient Education
- Protect medication from direct light.
- Dilute parenteral dose to 50 mg/cc with sterile water.
- Monitor I&O; intake must support 1,500 cc/day output (3,000–4,000 cc/day).
- Monitor IV site (pain, redness, or swelling); temperature; urinalysis.
- Teach patient
  - to be cautious when driving or involved in potentially hazardous tasks.
  - that medication may cause photosensitivity.
  - to maintain good hydration (approximately 10 to 12 glasses of fluid each day).

# Sulfapyridine

**Actions**
Antibacterial, anti-infective

**Uses**
Dermatitis (herpetiformis)

**Contraindications**
Hypersensitivity. *Use with caution:* Diabetes.

**Interactions**
Chlorpropamide, methotrexate, phenylbutazone, phenytoin, probenecid, salicylates, tolbutamide, warfarin

**Dose**
*Adult*  Initial dose, 500 mg qid; upon improvement, decrease 500 mg/day at 3-day intervals until a symptom-free status is achieved

**Forms**
Tablets

**Adverse Effects**
Crystalluria, drowsiness, headache, hematuria, nausea, urticaria, vomiting

## Special Nursing Considerations and Patient Education
- Protect medication from direct light.
- Monitor I&O, intake must support 1,500 cc/day output (3,000–4,000 cc/day).
- Monitor temperature, urinary pH.
- Be aware that
  - toxicity is common.
- Teach patient
  - to be cautious when driving or involved in potentially hazardous tasks.
  - that medication may cause photosensitivity.
  - to not take nonprescription medications without contacting physician first.
  - to maintain good hydration (approximately 10 to 12 glasses of fluid each day).

# Sulfisoxazole

**Brand Name**
　Gantrisin

**Actions**
　Antimicrobial; hinders folic acid formation in
　susceptible microorganisms

**Uses**
　Infections (ophthalmic, topical, urinary tract)

**Contraindications**
*Meds* Alcohol, multi-vitamins with p-amino benzoic
　　acid, urinary acidifiers
*Other* Group A beta-hemolytic streptococcal
　　infections. *Use with caution:* Acute
　　intermittent porphyria, allergies (general,
　　sulfonamides), anemia, dehydrogenase
　　deficiency, diabetes, hepatic or renal disease

**Interactions**
　Acetazolamide, aminobenzoic acid,
　chlorpropamide, hypoglycemics, methenamine,
　methotrexate, oral anticoagulants or antidiabetics,
　oxyphenbutazone, para-aminosalicylic acid,
　paraldehyde, penicillin, phenylbutazone, phenytoin,
　probenecid, urinary alkalinizing agents

**Dose**
*Adult* PO: initial dose, 2–4 gm; then 2–4 gm/day in
　　divided doses; *maximum* dose: 8 gm/day
*Peds* Over 2 months of age: initial dose, 75
　　mg/kg/day PO; *maintenance* dose: 150
　　mg/kg/day in 4–6 divided doses

## Forms
Emulsion, injection, ointment, pediatric
suspension, solutions, suppositories, syrup,
tablets, vaginal cream

## Adverse Effects
Crystalluria, diarrhea, headache, hematuria,
nausea, proteinuria, vomiting

## Special Nursing Considerations
## and Patient Education
- Protect medication from direct light.
- When administering IM, inject no more than 5
  cc/site.
- When administering IV, use sterile distilled water;
  do not mix with parenteral fluids.
- Monitor I&O; intake must support 1,500 cc/day
  output (3,000–4,000 cc/day).
- Monitor temperature, urinary pH; monitor diabetic
  patients for hypoglycemia.
- Teach patient
  - that medication may cause photosensitivity.
  - to take after eating to decrease GI irritation.
  - to maintain good hydration (approximately 10–12
    glasses of fluid each day).
  - to notify physician for hematuria, rash, sore
    throat.
  - to not take nonprescription medications without
    contacting physician first.

# Terbutaline Sulfate

## Brand Name
Brethine, Bricanyl

## Actions
Bronchodilator, sympathomimetic; relaxation of bronchial muscles and peripheral vasculature. Onset evident: SC 15 minutes.

## Uses
Bronchial asthma, bronchitis, emphysema, reversible bronchospasm

## Contraindications
MAO inhibitors, non-prescription antiasthmatics, propranolol, sympathomimetics. *Use with caution:* Diabetes, dysrhythmias, hypertension, hyperthyroidism, seizures

## Interactions
Antihistamines, antihypertensives, sodium levothyroxine, tricyclic antidepressants

## Dose
*Adult*  PO: 5 mg q6h; *maximum* dose: 15 mg/day
*Peds*  Adolescent: 2.5 mg tid PO; *maximum* dose: 7.5 mg/day PO

## Forms
Injection, tablets

## Adverse Effects
Blood pressure alterations, dizziness, drowsiness, headache, muscle cramps, nausea, nervousness, palpitations, tachycardia, tremors, vomiting

**Special Nursing Considerations
and Patient Education**
- Administer SC into lateral deltoid.
- Monitor blood pressure; take blood pressure and
  pulse before giving SC dose and compare with
  patient's guidelines.
- Teach patient to
  - be cautious when driving or involved in
    potentially hazardous tasks.
  - not use nonprescription inhalers.
  - notify physician if medication does not improve
    breathing within 15 minutes of administering
    medication.

# Tetracycline

**Brand Name**
Achromycin, Sumycin

**Actions**
Antiamoebic, antibacterial, antibiotic, antirickettsial; hinders protein synthesis in susceptible microorganisms

**Uses**
Granuloma inguinale, infections caused by gram negative and gram positive bacteria, lymphogranuloma, mycoplasma, ornithosis, psittacosis, rickettsial disease

**Contraindications**
*Meds* Antacids, antidiarrheals, dairy products, iron supplements, laxatives containing magnesium
*Other* History of hepatic disease; renal insufficiency. *Use with caution:* Hepatic or renal disease, lupus erythematosus

**Interactions**
Cephalosporins, methoxyflurane, oral anticoagulants, penicillins, sodium bicarbonate

**Dose**
*Adult* PO: 250 mg q6h; IM: 250–300 mg/day
*Peds* PO: 25–50 mg/kg/day; IM: 15–25 mg/kg/day

**Forms**
Capsules, injection, ointment, ophthalmic ointment, pediatric drops, suspension, syrup, tablets

**Adverse Effects**
Anorexia, diarrhea, dizziness, nausea, teeth discoloration (in patients under 8 years), vomiting

**Special Nursing Considerations
and Patient Education**
- Protect medication from light.
- Check expiration date prior to administration.
- Administer oral forms before meals or 2 hours after meals with a full glass of water.
- Administer IM dose deep into large muscle mass; give IV dose slowly.
- Monitor I&O, weight.
- Continue treatment 24–48 hours after temperature is normal.
- Be aware that
  - treatment for beta-hemolytic streptococci-group A infections continues for 10 days.
- Teach patient
  - that medication may cause photosensitivity.
  - to be cautious when driving or involved in potentially hazardous tasks.

# Theophylline

**Brand Name**
Tedral, Elixophyllin, Slo-Phyllin

**Actions**
Bronchodilator. Onset evident in 15–30 minutes.

**Uses**
Acute bronchial asthma

**Contraindications**
Peptic ulcer. *Use with caution:* Acute cardiac disease, cor pulmonale, glaucoma, gout, hepatic or renal disease, hypertension, hyperthyroidism, hypoxemia, myocardial damage, neonates, porphyria, prostatic hypertrophy

**Interactions**
Acetazolamide, allopurinol, anticoagulants, chlordiazepoxide, cimetidine, clindamycin, digitalis, erythromycin, furosemide, lincomycin, lithium, phenobarbital, phenytoin, propranolol, sympathomimetics

**Dose**
*Adult*  PO: 100–200 mg q6h
*Peds*  PO: 50–100 mg q6h

**Forms**
Capsules, injection, elixir, suppositories

**Adverse Effects**
Anorexia, dizziness, headache, insomnia, nausea, palpitations, restlessness, tachycardia, vomiting

## Special Nursing Considerations
## and Patient Education
- Administer medication 1 hour before or 2 hours after meals with a glass of water to decrease GI symptoms.
- Wait 4–6 hours when changing from IV to PO route.
- Monitor I&O, plasma levels, tolerance, vital signs.
- Be aware that
  - serum levels should be within 10–20 $\mu$/cc.
- Teach patient to
  - decrease caffeine intake because it potentiates medication.
  - be cautious when driving or involved in potentially hazardous tasks.
  - not take nonprescription medications without contacting physician.

# Thioridazine HCl

**Brand Name**
Mellaril

**Actions**
Antipsychotic, sedative; hinders dopamine action.
Onset evident in 1 week.

**Uses**
Behavior problems in children, dementia,
psychosis

**Contraindications**
*Meds* Alcohol
*Other* Cardiac disease. *Use with caution:* Bone-
marrow depression, epilepsy, glaucoma,
hepatic impairment, parkinsonism, prostatic
hypertrophy, respiratory disorders, Reye's
syndrome, urinary retention

**Interactions**
Amphetamines, antidiarrheals, atropine-like
medications, barbiturates, CNS depressants,
guanethidine, narcotics, phenytoin, tricyclic
antidepressants

**Dose**
*Adult* Initial dose, 25–100 mg tid; *maximum* dose:
800 mg/day; *maintenance* dose: 20–200 mg/day
*Peds* Over 2 yr: 0.5–3 mg/kg/day

**Forms**
Concentrate, tablets

**Adverse Effects**
Blurred vision, hypotension, impotence, nausea,
sedation, vomiting

**Special Nursing Considerations and Patient Education**
- Protect liquid form of medication from light.
- Dilute concentrate form per manufacturer's instructions.
- Monitor patient to ensure medication is swallowed.
- When discontinued, decrease dosage gradually.
- Teach patient
  - to be cautious when driving or involved in potentially hazardous tasks.
  - to use caution in hot weather and during strenuous exercise because of potential orthostatic hypotension.
  - to change position slowly to decrease hypotension.

# Thiothixene HCl

### Brand Name
Navane

### Actions
Antipsychotic, tranquilizer; depression of brainstem. Onset evident in 3 weeks.

### Uses
Acute or chronic schizophrenia

### Contraindications
*Meds* Alcohol, CNS depressants
*Other* Blood disorders, children under 12, parkinsonism. *Use with caution:* Cardiovascular disease, epilepsy, glaucoma, hepatic or renal disease, hypertension, peptic ulcer, prostatic hypertrophy, respiratory disorders, Reye's syndrome

### Interactions
Amphetamines, antidiarrheals, atropine-like medications, barbiturates, CNS depressants, guanethidine, narcotics, phenytoin, tricyclic antidepressants

### Dose
*Adult* PO: 2–5 mg bid–tid; parenteral: 4 mg bid–qid; *maximum* dose: 60 mg/day

### Forms
Capsules, concentrate, injection

### Adverse Effects
Blurred vision, constipation, dizziness, drowsiness, dry mouth, extrapyramidal symptoms, hypotension, insomnia

## Special Nursing Considerations and Patient Education

- Protect medication from direct light.
- Dilute concentrate form per manufacturer's instructions.
- Avoid contacting medication with hands because of possibility of contact dermatitis.
- When discontinued, decrease dosage gradually.
- Administer IM slowly into deep muscles; have patient remain recumbent for ½ hour after administration because of potential orthostatic hypotension.
- Monitor for fine vermicular tongue movements (may indicate early tardive dyskinesia).
- Offer hard candy (regular or sugar-free) to relieve dry mouth.
- Teach patient
  - to change position slowly to decrease hypotension.
  - that medication may cause photosensitivity.
  - to be cautious when driving or involved in potentially hazardous tasks.
  - notify physician for hemorrhage, jaundice, rash, sore throat, tremors, vision impairment, weakness.

# Thyroglobulin

**Brand Name**
Proloid

**Actions**
Thyroid hormone preparation; regulates cellular oxidation rate

**Uses**
Hypothyroidism

**Contraindications**
Hypopituitarism, uncorrected adrenal insufficiency. *Use with caution:* Arteriosclerosis, cardiac disease, congestive heart failure, coronary artery disease, diabetes, history of or current angina pectoris, hypertension, hyperthyroidism, MI, myxedema, renal dysfunction, thyrotoxicosis

**Interactions**
Antidiabetics, cholestyramine, insulin, ketamine, oral anticoagulants, phenytoin, sympathomimetics, tricyclic antidepressants

**Dose**
*Adult* Individualized; initial dose, 15–60 mg; *maintenance* dose: 32–200 mg/day
*Peds* Individualized; 2–60 mg/day

**Forms**
Tablets

**Adverse Effects**
Angina, dysrhythmias, headache, hyperthyroidism, nervousness, palpitations, sweating

## Special Nursing Considerations and Patient Education

- Protect medication from direct light.
- Take pulse prior to administration; hold if less than 100.
- Administer medication as one dose before breakfast.
- Continue medication as directed.
- Be aware
  - that transfer to and from sodium liothyronin should occur gradually to prevent relapse.

# Ticarcillin Disodium

**Brand Name**
  Ticar

**Actions**
  Antibacterial, antibiotic, anti-infective; hinders
  synthesis of cell walls in susceptible
  microorganisms

**Uses**
  Gram-negative, genitourinary tract infections

**Contraindications**
  Allergy to penicillin. *Use with caution:* General
  allergies, hepatic or renal impairment

**Interactions**
  Erythromycin, gentamicin*, probenecid,
  tetracycline, tobramycin*
    *These are synergistic against Pseudomonas,
    but must be infused at least 1 hour apart.

**Dose**
*Adult* 150–300 mg/kg/day in divided doses
*Peds* Neonates under 2,000 gm: initial dose, 100
    mg/kg; then 75 mg/kg q8h during 1st week of
    age; age 8 days and over: 100 mg/kg q4h

**Forms**
  Injection

**Adverse Effects**
  Dermatitis, diarrhea, hypernatremia, hypokalemia,
  nausea, neuromuscular excitability, neurotoxicity,
  pruritus, superinfections, vomiting

**Special Nursing Considerations
and Patient Education**
- Administer IV dose per manufacturer's
  instructions.
- Administer IM dose with no more than 2 cc/site; for
  adult, inject into upper, outer quadrant of buttocks
  or midlateral thigh; for children, into midlateral
  thigh.
- Keep out-patient in clinic for 30 minutes after
  receiving injection in case of allergic reaction.
- Monitor I&O.
- Be alert to indications of hypernatremia and
  hypokalemia (see Appendix B).

# Tolazamide

**Brand Name**
Tolinase

**Actions**
Hypoglycemic

**Uses**
Diabetes (stable, uncontrolled by diet)

**Contraindications**
*Meds* Alcohol
*Other* Complicated, diet-controlled, or juvenile
diabetes; hepatic or renal impairment;
infection; surgery; trauma. *Use with caution:*
Acidosis, burns, diabetic coma, fever, hepatic
impairment, ketoacidosis, ketosis, nausea,
peptic ulcer, porphyria, severe infection,
surgery, thyroid and renal dysfunction,
trauma, vomiting

**Interactions**
Anti-inflammatories, barbiturates, bishydroxy-
coumarin, chloramphenicol, chlorpromazine,
clofibrate, coumarin anticoagulants, dextrothyroxine, epinephrine, estrogens, guanethidine,
hypnotics, insulin, isoniazid, MAO inhibitors,
nicotinic acid, oral contraceptives, oxyphenbutazone, oxytetracycline, phenylbutazone,
phenytamidol, phenytoin, probenecid, propranolol,
pyrazinamide, salicylates, sedatives, sulfa-
phenazole, sulfisoxazole, sulfonamides,
thiazide diuretics

**Dose**
*Adult* Individualized; 100 mg–1 gm in 1–2 divided
doses/day

**Forms**
Tablets

**Adverse Effects**
Anorexia, constipation, diarrhea, headache, hepatic toxicities, hypoglycemia, nausea, vomiting

**Special Nursing Considerations and Patient Education**
- Monitor for hypoglycemia, weight.
- Teach patient
  - about prescribed diet and how to follow it.
  - to be cautious when driving or involved in potentially hazardous tasks.
  - that medication may cause photosensitivity and urine may darken.
  - to carry some type of Medic Alert card or bracelet.
  - to see physician once weekly for first six weeks of use.
  - to check urine daily for sugar and acetone.
  - to notify physician if becomes ill.

# Tolbutamide

**Brand Name**
Orinase

**Actions**
Hypoglycemic. Onset evident in 3–6 hours.

**Uses**
Diabetes, diagnostic test for pancreatic islet cell tumors

**Contraindications**
*Meds* Alcohol
*Other* Acidosis; burns; complicated, diet-controlled, or juvenile diabetes; hepatic or renal insufficiency; ketoacidosis; ketosis. *Use with caution:* Nausea, peptic ulcer, porphyria, thyroid dysfunction, vomiting

**Interactions**
Anabolic steroids, anti-inflammatories, barbiturates, chloramphenicol, chlorpromazine, corticosteroids, cortisone, coumarin anti-coagulants, epinephrine, estrogens, ethacrynic acid, furosemide, hypnotics, isoniazid, MAO inhibitors, nicotinic acid, oral contraceptives, phenylbutazone, probenecid, propanolol, pyrazinamide, salicylates, sedatives, sulfin-pyrazone, sulfisoxazole, sulfonamides, thiazide diuretics, thyroid preparations

**Dose**
*Adult* 1–2 gm/day; *maintenance* dose: 0.25–2 gm/day

**Forms**
Tablets

## Adverse Effects

Anorexia, constipation, diarrhea, headache, hepatic toxicity, hypoglycemia, nausea, pruritus, vomiting

## Special Nursing Considerations and Patient Education

- Monitor for hypoglycemia, urine tests (acetone and sugar), weight.
- Teach patient
  - that medication may cause breath to be sweet-smelling.
  - that medication may cause photosensitivity.
  - to check urine daily for sugar and acetone.
  - to follow prescribed diet.
  - to carry some type of Medic Alert card or bracelet.
  - to not take any new medications without contacting physician first.
  - to be cautious when driving or involved in potentially hazardous tasks.
  - to notify physician of indications of hypoglycemia (e.g., drowsiness, fatigue, headache).
  - to carry source of glucose (e.g., candy).
  - notify physician for ecchymosis, fever, jaundice, rash, sore throat.

# Tranylcypromine Sulfate

**Brand Name**
  Parnate

**Actions**
  Antidepressant, MAO inhibitor. Onset evident in
  2–3 weeks.

**Uses**
  Endogenous or reactive depression, involutional
  melancholia

**Contraindications**
*Meds* Alcohol, CNS depressants, sympathomimetics
*Other* Arteriosclerosis, atony colitis, cardiovascular
  or cerebrovascular disorders, children under 16,
  elderly, epilepsy, hepatic or renal impairment,
  hypernatremia, hypertension, hyperthyroid,
  paranoid schizophrenia, pheochromocytoma.
  *Use with caution:* Diabetes, edema, glaucoma,
  hypoglycemia, jaundice, visual impairment

**Interactions**
  Anesthetics, antihypertensives, antiparkinsonism,
  barbiturates, guanethidine, oral antidiabetics,
  reserpine, tricyclic antidepressants

**Dose**
*Adult* Initial dose: 10 mg bid x 2 weeks; *maintenance*
  dose: 10–20 mg/day; *maximum* dose: 30 mg/day

**Forms**
  Tablets

**Adverse Effects**
  Anorexia, confusion, constipation, dizziness, dry
  mouth, edema, headache, hypertensive crisis,
  hypotension, insomnia, nausea, tremors, vomiting

**Special Nursing Considerations
and Patient Education**
- Protect medication from heat and light.
- Take blood pressure prior to beginning of
  treatment.
- Use caution when administering to a patient with
  suicidal potential; ensure patient swallows dose.
- Offer hard candy (regular or sugar-free) to relieve
  dry mouth.
- Monitor blood pressure, I&O, weight.
- Discontinue gradually; rapid withdrawal can cause
  side effects.
- Be aware that
  - this medication is more likely to cause
    hypertensive crisis than other MAO inhibitors.
- Teach patient
  - that medication may cause photophobia.
  - to not take any other medications without
    contacting physician first.
  - to avoid foods containing tryptophan or tyramine
    (see Appendix F).
  - to change position slowly to decrease
    hypotension.
  - to be cautious when driving or involved in
    potentially hazardous tasks.
  - to use caution during strenuous exercise
    because of its impact on blood pressure.
  - notify physician for chest pain, neck stiffening,
    pupil dilation, vomiting.
  - Monitor for indications of hypertensive crisis
    (e.g., nausea, occipital headache, palpitations,
    perspiring); notify physician if any occur.

# Trazodone HCl

**Brand Name**
Desyrel

**Actions**
Antidepressant. Onset evident in 1–4 weeks.

**Uses**
Depression

**Contraindications**
*Meds* Anesthetics
*Other* Children, ECT, MI (initial recovery phase). *Use with caution:* Cardiovascular disease

**Interactions**
Alcohol, antihypertensives, barbiturates, CNS depressants, MAO inhibitors

**Dose**
*Adult* Initial dose: 150 mg/day; may be increased by 50 mg/day q3–4d; *maximum* dose: inpatient 600 mg/day, outpatient 400 mg/day

**Forms**
Tablets

**Adverse Effects**
Blurred vision, confusion, constipation, dizziness, drowsiness, dry mouth, fatigue, hallucinations, headache, hypotension, incoordination, insomnia, nausea, nervousness, vomiting

**Special Nursing Considerations
and Patient Education**
- Administer with or shortly after meals to decrease GI irritation.
- Use caution when administering to a patient with suicidal potential; ensure patient swallows dose.
- Offer hard candy (regular or sugar free) to relieve dry mouth.
- Teach patient
  - to be cautious when driving or involved in potentially hazardous tasks.

# Triamterene

**Brand Name**
Dyazide, Dyrenium

**Actions**
Antihypertensive, potassium-sparing diuretic; hinders reabsorption of sodium in distal tubule. Onset evident in 2–4 hours.

**Uses**
Edema caused by cirrhosis, congestive heart failure, or hyperaldosteronism; idiopathic or steroid-induced edema

**Contraindications**
*Meds* Lithium, spironolactone
*Other* Anuria, hepatic disease, hyperkalemia, renal disorders. *Use with caution:* Diabetes, gout

**Interactions**
Antihypertensives, digitalis, diuretics, methotrexate, oral antidiabetics

**Dose**
*Adult* Individualized; 100 mg bid; *maximum* dose: 300 mg/day
*Peds* Individualized; 2–4 mg/kg/day in divided doses

**Forms**
Capsules

**Adverse Effects**
Diarrhea, dizziness, electrolyte imbalance, headache, hyperkalemia, hyponatremia, nausea, vomiting, weakness

## Special Nursing Considerations and Patient Education
- Protect medication from direct light.
- Monitor BP during dosage adjustment; monitor I&O, weight.
- Administer medication after meals to decrease GI distress.
- When discontinued, decrease dosage gradually to prevent rebound kaliuresis.
- Teach patient
  - to avoid potassium-rich foods and salt substitutes (see Appendix F).
  - that medication may cause photosensitivity, and may color urine blue.
  - to be cautious when driving or involved in potentially hazardous tasks.
  - to notify physician for signs and symptoms of hyperkalemia, hyponatremia (see Appendix B).

# Trifluoperazine HCl

**Brand Name**
  Stelazine

**Actions**
  Antipsychotic, tranquilizer. Onset evident in 1–2
  hours.

**Uses**
  Schizophrenia

**Contraindications**
*Meds* Alcohol
*Other* Blood disorders, bone-marrow disorders,
      children under 16 unless hospitalized, hepatic
      impairment. *Use with caution:* Angina, epilepsy,
      glaucoma, parkinsonism, peptic ulcer,
      prostatic hypertrophy, respiratory disorder

**Interactions**
  Amphetamines, antacids, anticonvulsants,
  antidepressants, antidiarrheals, antihistamine,
  atropine-like medications, CNS depressants,
  guanethidine, hypnotics, levodopa, MAO inhibitors,
  narcotics, phenytoin, quinidine, sedatives.

**Dose**
*Adult* PO: Initial dose: 1–5 mg bid; usual dose: 15–20
      mg/day; *maximum* dose: 40 mg/day
*Peds* PO: 6–12 yr (hospitalized): 1 mg qd–bid

**Forms**
  Concentrate, injection, tablets

**Adverse Effects**
  Agitation, blurred vision, constipation, dizziness,
  drowsiness, dry mouth, extrapyramidal symptoms,
  hypotension, nasal congestion, tachycardia

**Special Nursing Considerations
and Patient Education**
- Protect medication from direct light.
- Dilute concentrate per manufacturer's instructions.
- Administer IM dose slowly into large muscle mass;
  keep patient in recumbent position for ½ hour
  after administration.
- Monitor for fine vermicular tongue movements
  (may indicate early tardive dyskinesia).
- Offer hard candy (regular or sugar-free) to relieve
  dry mouth.
- When discontinued, decrease dosage gradually.
- Teach patient
  - that medication may cause photosensitivity and
    may discolor urine.
  - to be cautious when driving or involved in
    potentially hazardous tasks.
  - to use caution in hot weather and during
    strenuous exercise because of their impact on
    circulation.

# Trifluridine

**Brand Name**
Viroptic

**Actions**
Antiviral; hinders synthesis of DNA in
mammalian cells

**Uses**
Infections not responding to idoxuridine and
vidarabine, primary keratoconjunctivitis, recurrent
epithelial keratitis due to herpes simplex virus 1
and 2

**Contraindications**
Hypersensitivity

**Interactions**
Glaucoma

**Dose**
*Adult*  1 gtt to affected eye q2h while awake;
*maximum* dose: 9 gtt until ulcer reepithetial-
ized, then 1 gtt q4h while awake for a
*minimum* of 7 days

**Forms**
Ophthalmic solution

**Adverse Effects**
Epithelial keratopathy, intraocular pressure
increase, keratitis sicca, palpebral edema,
superficial punctate keratopathy

**Special Nursing Considerations
and Patient Education**
- Take care to not contaminate tip of dropper.
- Teach patient to
  - notify physician if no improvement occurs after
    7 days or complete healing does not occur after
    14 days.

# Trihexyphenidyl HCl

**Brand Name**
Artane

**Actions**
Anticholinergic, antidyskinetic, muscle relaxant; affects parasympathetic system. Onset evident in 1 hour.

**Uses**
Extrapyramidal disorders from CNS medications, parkinsonism

**Contraindications**
Arteriosclerosis, children. *Use with caution:* Glaucoma, myasthenia gravis, obstructive disease of the GU or GI tract, prostatic hypertrophy

**Interactions**
Alcohol, antacids, antidiarrheals, antihistamines, antimuscarinics, barbiturates, CNS depressants, haloperidol, MAO inhibitors, phenothiazines, primidone, procainamide, quinidine, tricyclic antidepressants

**Dose**
*Adult* Individualized; initial dose: 1 mg/day; increase to 6–10 mg/day in divided doses

**Forms**
Elixir, sustained-release capsules, tablets

**Adverse Effects**
Blurred vision, constipation, dizziness, drowsiness, dry mouth, insomnia, nausea, nervousness, urinary retention

**Special Nursing Considerations
and Patient Education**
- Protect medication from direct light.
- Monitor vital signs until dosage is adjusted.
- Offer hard candy (regular or sugar-free) to relieve dry mouth.
- When discontinued, decrease dosage gradually.
- Be aware that
  - tolerance can develop.
- Teach patient to
  - take with meals to decrease gastric upset.
  - not take any nonprescription cough or hay fever preparations.
  - be cautious when driving or involved in potentially hazardous tasks.
  - use caution in hot weather and during strenuous exercise as medication may suppress perspiration.
  - increase fluid and bulk intake to decrease constipation.
  - notify physician for eye pain

# Trimethobenzamide HCl

**Brand Name**
Tigan

**Actions**
Antiemetic; inhibits medulla's chemoreceptor trigger zone. Onset evident in 20–40 minutes.

**Uses**
Nausea, vomiting

**Contraindications**
*Meds* Alcohol, CNS depressants
*Other* Benzocaine hypersensitivity, children (IM route), CNS depression, neonates and premature infants (suppositories). *Use with caution:* Allergies to antihistamines, dehydration, electrolyte imbalance, encephalitides, fever, gastroenteritis, Reye's syndrome

**Interactions**
Alkaloids derived from belladonna, barbiturates, phenothiazines, sedatives

**Dose**
*Adult* PO: 250 mg tid–qid
*Peds* Under 66 kg: (PO, rectal), 100 mg tid–qid
66–198 kg: (PO, rectal) 100–200 mg tid–qid

**Forms**
Capsules, injection, pediatric suppositories, suppositories, tablets

**Adverse Effects**
Blurred vision, depression, diarrhea, disorientation, dizziness, drowsiness, dry mouth, extrapyramidal symptoms, headache, hypotension, jaundice, muscle cramps

## Special Nursing Considerations and Patient Education

- Administer IM dose deep in upper, outer quadrant of gluteal muscle.
- Monitor blood pressure per physician's guidelines.
- Store suppositories in refrigerator.
- Be aware that
  - medication is administered to children only for prolonged vomiting with unknown etiology.
  - medication may mask toxic levels of other medications.
- Teach patient to
  - change position slowly to decrease hypotension.
  - be cautious when driving or involved in potentially hazardous tasks.
  - notify physician for rash.

# Tybamate

**Brand Name**
Tybatran

**Actions**
Antianxiety, tranquilizer. Onset evident in 30 minutes–2 hours.

**Uses**
Anxiety, tension

**Contraindications**
*Meds* Alcohol, CNS depressants
*Other* Children under 6, history of acute intermittent porphyria. *Use with caution:* Convulsive disorders, epilepsy, hepatic or renal impairment

**Interactions**
Anticonvulsants, antidepressants, hypnotics, MAO inhibitors, narcotics, phenothiazines, sedatives, tranquilizers

**Dose**
*Adult* 250–500 mg tid–qid; *maximum* dose: 3 gm/day
*Peds* 6 yr or older: 20–35 mg/kg/day in 3–4 divided doses

**Forms**
Capsules

**Adverse Effects**
Ataxia, blurred vision, confusion, dizziness, drowsiness, dry mouth, feeling of unreality, glossitis, grand mal seizures, headache, hypotension, light-headedness, nausea, weakness

**Special Nursing Considerations
and Patient Education**
- Encourage patient to verbalize feelings of anxiety.
- Offer hard candy (regular or sugar-free) to relieve dry mouth.
- When discontinued, decrease dosage gradually to prevent withdrawal symptoms.
- Teach patient to
  - be cautious when driving or involved in potentially hazardous tasks.
  - decrease caffeine intake because of its stimulant effect.

# Undecylenic Acid/ Zinc Undecylenate

**Brand Name**
  Desenex

**Actions**
  Antifungal

**Uses**
  Athlete's feet, ringworm

**Contraindications**
  Hypersensitivity. *Use with caution:* Circulatory impairment, diabetes

**Interactions**
  None

**Dose**
*Adult*  Apply topically bid
*Peds*  Same as adult

**Forms**
  Ointment, powder, soap, solution

**Adverse Effects**
  None

**Special Nursing Considerations
and Patient Education**
- Teach patient
  - to not use medication near eyes.
  - regarding correct hygiene for feet.

# Vasopressin

**Brand Name**
Pitressin Tannate

**Actions**
Antidiuretic, posterior pituitary hormone, vasoconstrictor; aids in reabsorption of water in renal nephrons

**Uses**
Diabetes insipidus, gaseous distention

**Contraindications**
Angina, arteriosclerosis, chronic nephritis with nitrogen retention, ischemic heart disease, PVCs; IV route. *Use with caution:* Asthma, cardiac failure, children, migraine headache, vascular disease

**Interactions**
Acetaminophin, antidiabetic agents, diuretics, gangleonic blocking agents, heparin, lithium

**Dose**
*Adult* Individualized; IM, SC 5–10 U 2–8x/day
*Peds* Individualized

**Forms**
Injection

**Adverse Effects**
Circumoral pallor, dysrhythmias, hypersensitivity, MI, water intoxication

## Special Nursing Considerations and Patient Education

- Before giving first dose, establish baseline data on patient's alertness, blood pressure, orientation, I&O, weight; recheck periodically throughout therapy.
- Monitor specific gravity and serum osmolality of patient's urine.
- Teach patient
  - to monitor urine specific gravity and serum osmolality at home per physician's guidelines.

# Verapamil HCl

## Brand Name
Calan, Isoptin

## Actions
Antidysrhythmic, calcium antagonist; hinders calcium movement into select cardiovascular cells. Onset evident: IV 2–5 minutes.

## Uses
Paroxysmal supraventricular tachycardia, Prinzmetal's angina pectoris

## Contraindications
*Meds* Beta-adrenergic blocking medications (given IV), calcium, disopyramide

*Other* Cardiogenic shock, 2nd or 3nd degree AV block, severe congestive heart failure, severe hypotension

## Interactions
Antihypertensives, digitalis, highly protein-bound medications, quinidine

## Dose
*Adult* IV bolus: initial dose, 5–10 mg; 10 mg 30 minutes later; PO 240–480 mg/day in divided doses

*Peds* Under 1 yr: 0.1–0.2 mg/kg over 2 min 1–15 yr: 0.1–0.3 mg/kg over 2 min; repeat dose after 30 min if necessary; *maximum* single dose 10 mg

## Forms
Solution (injection), tablets

## Adverse Effects
Bradycardia, constipation, dizziness, edema, headache, hypotension, nausea, tachycardia

## Special Nursing Considerations and Patient Education

- Monitor blood pressure before and after giving medication to evaluate patient's response.
- Monitor via a cardiac monitor during IV administration.
- Keep emergency equipment readily available.
- Monitor I&O.
- Teach patient
  - to change position slowly to decrease hypotension.
  - to be cautious when driving or involved in potentially hazardous tasks.

# Warfarin Sodium

**Brand Name**
Coumadin, Panwarfin

**Actions**
Anticoagulant; hinders synthesis of prothrombin. Onset evident in 12 hours.

**Uses**
Adjunct for coronary occlusion; atrial fibrillation with embolization, prophylactic use in pulmonary or venous thrombosis

**Contraindications**

*Meds* Alcohol, anesthetics

*Other* Blood dyscrasias, hemorrhagic tendency, hepatic or renal disease, malignant hypertension, peptic ulcer, polyarthritis, surgery, threatened abortion, ulcerative colitis, vitamin C deficiency. *Use with caution:* Allergies, anaphylactic disorders, diabetes, hepatic or renal insufficiency, infectious diseases, moderate to severe hypertension, polycythemia vera, vitamin K deficiency

**Interactions**
Allopurinol, anabolic drugs, androgenic anabolic steroids, androgens, antacids, antibiotics, antidepressants, antihistamines, barbiturates, benzodiazepines, carbamazepine, chloral hydrate, chloramphenicol, chlorpromazine, cholestyramine, cortisone, coumarin, digitalis, disulfiram, d-thyroxine, estrogens, ethacrynic acid, glucagon, glutethimide, griseofulvin, haloperidol, hydroxyzine, indomethacin, insulin, isoniazid, mefenamic acid, mercaptopurine, methyldopa,

methylphenidate, nalidixic acid, nortriptyline, oral
contraceptives, oxyphenbutazone, para-
aminosalicylic acid, phenylbutazone, phenyl-
propanolamine, phenyramidal, probenecid,
propylthiouracil, quinidine, reserpine, salicylates,
sulfinpyrazone, sulfonamides, sulfonylureas,
thyroid preparations, tolbutamide
NOTE: Oral anticoagulants have a greater potential
for significant interactions than any other class of
drugs.

## Dose
*Adult*    PO: initial dose, 40–60 mg, depending upon
prothrombin times; *maintenance* dose: 2–10
mg/day depending upon prothrombin times

## Forms
Injection, tablets

## Adverse Effects
Abdominal cramps, anorexia, dermatitis, diarrhea,
hemorrhage, nausea, urticaria, vomiting

## Special Nursing Considerations
and Patient Education
• Protect medication from direct light.
• Administer medications exactly as ordered.
• Administer as a single daily dose unless ordered
  otherwise.
• Monitor prothrombin times.
• Do not change patient's diet because of possible
  impact on drug's effectiveness.
• When discontinued, decrease dosage gradually.

*(continued)*

# Warfarin Sodium (continued)

- Teach patient
  - that medication may discolor urine to orange.
  - to carry some type of Medic Alert card or bracelet.
  - to not take any other medications without notifying physician.
  - to notify physician if becomes ill or shows any signs of hemorrhage.
  - to use soft toothbrush and electric razor to decrease possibility of hemorrhage.
  - if having dental work done, to inform dentist about this medication.

# Part II
# Appendices

# Appendix A
# Abbreviations

| | |
|---|---|
| ACTH | Adrenocorticotropic hormone |
| AC | Before meals |
| AM | Morning |
| amps | Ampules |
| APTT | Activated partial thromboplastin time |
| ASAP | As soon as possible |
| AV | Atrioventricular |
| Avg. | Average |
| BID | Twice a day |
| BUN | Blood urea nitrogen |
| CBC | Complete blood count |
| cc | Cubic centimeter |
| cm² | Square centimeter |
| CNS | Central nervous system |
| CVA | Cerebral vascular accident |
| CVP | Central venous pressure |
| d | Day |
| D/C | Discontinue |
| DNA | Deoxyribonucleic acid |
| ECT | Electric convulsion therapy |
| EKG | Electrocardiogram |
| GI | Gastrointestinal |
| gm | Gram |
| gtt | Drops |
| GU | Genitourinary |
| h | Hour |
| hs | Hour of sleep |
| IM | Intramuscular |
| I&O | Intake and output |
| IV | Intravenous |
| KCl | Potassium chloride |

| kg | Kilogram |
| kg/min | Kilogram per minute |
| $m^2$ | Square meter |
| MAO | Monoamine oxidase (MAO inhibitor) |
| Mg | Magnesium |
| $\mu g$ | Microgram |
| mg | Milligram |
| MI | Myocardial infarction |
| min | Minute |
| ml | Milliliter |
| $mm^3$ | Cubic millimeter |
| PO | By mouth |
| pc | After meals |
| PM | Afternoon |
| prn | As needed |
| PTT | Partial thromboplastin time |
| PVC | Premature ventricular contraction |
| q | Every |
| qd | Every day |
| qid | Four times a day |
| qod | Every other day |
| RNA | Ribonucleic acid |
| SC | Subcutaneous |
| tid | Three times a day |
| U | Units |
| WBC | White blood cells |
| x | Times |
| yr | Year |

# Appendix B
# Side Effect Groupings

*Allergic reactions*
- Delayed: angioedema, arthralgia, fever, lymph-adenopathy, splenomegaly
- Mild: angioedema, asthma, cramping (abdominal), diarrhea, dizziness, drowsiness, dyspepsia, fever, headache, hives, nausea, pruritis, rash, rhinitis, tinnitus, vomiting
- Severe: bone-marrow depression, confusion, extrapyramidal symptoms, fatigue, high fever, hallucinations, hemorrhage, hepatitis, jaundice, joint pains, palpitations, sore throat, weakness

*Androgenic effects:* breast-size reduction, hirsutism, voice deepening

*Drug fever:* ataxia, blurred vision, dizziness, irritability, numbness and tingling (circumoral/peripheral), weakness

*Ergotism:* confusion, diarrhea, dizziness, headache, nausea, vomiting

*Extrapyramidal symptoms:* akathisia, dystonia, parkinsonism, tardive dyskinesia

*Hyperglycemia:* excessive hunger and thirst, excessive urination, headache, nausea, positive urinary glucose and ketones, pulse increase, sweet-smelling breath, weight loss

*Hyperkalemia:* areflexia, breathing difficulty, confusion, parethesias, weakness

*Hypoglycemia:* anxiety, diaphoresis, drowsiness, fatigue, headache, lassitude, nausea, tremulousness

*Hypokalemia:* anorexia, confusion, hypotension, lethargy, muscle weakness, nausea

*Hyponatremia:* abdominal cramps, drowsiness, dry mouth, lethargy, thirst

*Hypertensive crisis:* increasing confusion, rapid increase in blood pressure, vision changes

*Lupus erythematosus syndrome:* arthritis, fever, myalgia, pleuritic pain, polyarthralgia, skin lesions

*Nephrotoxicity:* albuminuria, hematuria, retention of nitrogen, urinary casts

*Ototoxicity:* deafness, dizziness, sense of fullness in the ears, tinnitus, vertigo

*Renal failure:* albuminuria, azotemia, cylinduria

*Thrombosis:* chest/leg pain, respiratory distress

*Uremia:* drowsiness, foul breath, headache, lethargy, restlessness, vomiting

# Appendix C
# Nursing Interventions for
# Common Side Effects

*Bone-marrow suppression*
- Observe for signs and symptoms of infection, i.e., slow healing wound with inflammation, swelling and/or discharge or a cold that does not get better.
- Observe any abnormal bleeding tendencies: i.e., increased bruising, petechiae, frequent nose-bleeds, bleeding from gums.
- Brush teeth with toothettes or clean with gauze; avoid hard toothbrushes.
- Apply pressure for several minutes over injection sites.
- Observe changes in activity level and physical appearance for anemia, i.e., lethargy, fatigability, pallor of the skin and mucous membranes, dyspnea, heart palpitations.


*Constipation*
- Increase intake of foods high in fiber.
- Increase intake of water and other fluids.
- Include more fresh vegetables and fruits in the diet.
- Do not utilize laxatives unless directed to do so by the physician.

*Nausea*
- Keep dry carbohydrate foods at the bedside (dry crackers or toast). Eat a small amount before getting out of bed.
- Eat small frequent meals rather than three large meals.
- Monitor diet and eliminate those foods that aggravate the nausea.
- Do not utilize medications unless directed to do so by the physician.

*Orthostatic hypotension*
- When the patient is getting out of bed:
  - Have a chair or other support near the bedside.
  - Sit up slowly.
  - Dangle legs and feet over the side of the bed for several minutes.
  - Slowly stand up, sitting down if any dizziness occurs.
- When the patient is standing up from a chair:
  - Move to the edge of the chair slowly.
  - Sit there for a few minutes.
  - Slowly stand up, sitting down if any dizziness occurs.
  - Utilize a side chair or other support to stand up.

# Appendix D
# Conversion Information

## APOTHECARY SYSTEM TO METRIC SYSTEM
## (WEIGHT)

| | | | | |
|---|---|---|---|---|
| gr xv | = 1.0 | gm = | 1000 | mg |
| gr x | = 0.6 | gm = | 600 | mg |
| gr viiss (ss = ½) | = 0.5 | gm = | 500 | mg |
| gr v | = 0.3 | gm = | 300 | mg |
| gr iii | = 0.2 | gm = | 200 | mg |
| gr 1-½ | = 0.1 | gm = | 100 | mg |
| gr 1 | = 0.06 | gm = | 60 | mg |
| gr ¾ | = 0.05 | gm = | 50 | mg |
| gr ½ | = 0.03 | gm = | 30 | mg |
| gr ¼ | = 0.015 | gm = | 15 | mg |
| gr ⅙ | = 0.010 | gm = | 10 | mg |
| gr ⅛ | = 0.008 | gm = | 8 | mg |
| gr 1/12 | = 0.005 | gm = | 5 | mg |
| gr 1/15 | = 0.004 | gm = | 4 | mg |
| gr 1/20 | = 0.0032 | gm = | 3 | mg |
| gr 1/30 | = 0.0022 | gm = | 2 | mg |
| gr 1/40 | = 0.0015 | gm = | 1.5 | mg |
| gr 1/50 | = 0.0012 | gm = | 1.2 | mg |
| gr 1/60 | = 0.001 | gm = | 1 | mg |
| gr 1/100 | = 0.0006 | gm = | 0.6 | mg |
| gr 1/120 | = 0.0005 | gm = | 0.5 | mg |
| gr 1/150 | = 0.0004 | gm = | 0.4 | mg |
| gr 1/200 | = 0.0003 | gm = | 0.3 | mg |
| gr 1/300 | = 0.0002 | gm = | 0.2 | mg |
| gr 1/600 | = 0.0001 | gm = | 0.1 | mg |

## METRIC SYSTEM TO APOTHECARY SYSTEM

### Weight

| | | | |
|---|---|---|---|
| 0.06 | gm | = 1 | grain |
| 1 | gm | = 15 | grains |
| 4 | gm | = 1 | dram |
| 30 | gr | = 1 | ounce |
| 1 | kg | = 2.2 | pounds |

### Volume

| | | | |
|---|---|---|---|
| 0.06 | ml | = 1 | minim |
| 1 | ml | = 15 | minims |
| 4 | ml | = 1 | fluidram |
| 30 | ml | = 1 | fluidounce |
| 500 | ml | = 1 | pint |
| 1000 | ml | = 1 | quart |

# Appendix E
# General Guidelines for the Administration of Medications

Exercise caution when administering any medication to:

- Children
- Debilitated individuals
- Drug dependent individuals
- Elderly individuals
- Lactating females
- Pregnant females
- Individuals anticipating immediate surgery

Exercise caution when administering any medication to an individual for the first time.

Administration of any medication to an individual who previously experienced an allergic or hypersensitive reaction is contraindicated.

Remind patients to

- Take medications exactly as directed.
- Check dates on all medications prior to taking.
- Not discontinue a medication without conferring with the physician.

Available information on a medication is not indicative of the level of safety for that medication.

Excretion of medication occurs through the intestines, kidneys, liver, lungs or skin, and impairment of these organs indicates the need for caution when administering medications.

Advise patients to complete the regimen of medications that has been ordered even if they no longer feel ill.

Crushing an enteric coated or sustained release capsule/tablet is contraindicated. Mixing the contents of sustained release capsules for administration is contraindicated.

Include discharge teaching for any medications which the patient will be taking at home.

Review the patient's current medications when administering a new medication to avoid any problematic interactions.

Advising patients to be "cautious" indicates that they will experience some impairment in their normal levels of functioning.

# Appendix F
# Food Groupings

- *Potassium-rich:* almonds, apricots, bananas, beans (lima, navy), beef, chicken, citrus fruits, coconut, dates, dried figs, fish, lentils, melons, milk, orange juice, peaches, peanut butter, raw carrots, rye crackers
- *Tyramine-rich:* avocados, bananas, beverages (from meat/yeast extracts), broad beans, caffeine, cheese, chicken, chocolate, figs, licorice, liver, meat tenderizer, pickled herring, raisins, sour cream, soy sauce, unpasteurized beer, vermouth, wine (chianti), yeast extracts, yogurt

# References

Adrenergics (sympathomimetics). (1983). *Nursing 83, 13*(1), 64a-64b.

Albanese, J. (1979). *Nurses' Drug Reference.* New York: McGraw-Hill.

Aminoglycosides. (1983). *Nursing 83, 13*(2), 64a-64b.

Antianxiety agents. (1983). *Nursing 83, 13*(4), 64a-64b.

Antihypertensives. (1983). *Nursing 83, 13*(3), 64a-64b.

Armstrong, M., Dickason, E., Howe, J., Jones, D., & Snider, M. (Eds.). (1979). *McGraw-Hill Handbook of Clinical Nursing.* New York: McGraw-Hill.

Bergersen, B. & Goth, A. (1977). *Pharmacology in Nursing,* 14th Ed. St. Louis: Mosby.

Brooks, S. (Ed.). (1978). *Nurses' Drug Reference.* Boston: Little, Brown.

Govoni, L. & Hayes, J. (1982). *Drugs & Nursing Implications.* New York: Appleton-Century-Crofts.

Hussar, D., PhD. (1982). New drugs. *Nursing 82, 12*(5), 34.

Kirilloff, L. & Libbals, S. (1983). Drugs for asthma: a complete guide. *American Journal of Nursing. 83,* 55-61.

Loebl, S., Spratto, G. & Heckheimer, E. (1980). *The Nurse's Drug Handbook,* (2nd ed.). New York: Wiley.

Long, J. (1977). *The Essential Guide to Prescription Drugs: What You Need to Know for Safe Drug Use.* New York: Harper & Row.

Nurses' drug alert. (1982). *American Journal of Nursing, 82*(7), 1121-1128.

Nurses' drug alert. (1982). *American Journal of Nursing, 82*(9), 1425-1432.

Nurses' drug alert. (1982). *American Journal of Nursing, 82*(11), 1749-1756.

*Nursing 81 Drug Handbook.* (1981). Horsham, PA: Intermed Communications.

Penicillins. (1983). *Nursing 83, 13*(6), 64a-64b.

Thrombolytic enzymes. (1983). *Nursing 83, 13*(5), 64a-64b.

*Physicians' Desk Reference.* (1984). (38th ed.). Oradell, NJ: Medical Economics Co.

US Pharmacopial Convention. (1980). *United States Dispensing Information 1980.* Easton, PA: Mack Printing Company.

Wiener, M., Pepper, A., Kuhn-Weisman, G., and Romano, J. (1979). *Clinical Pharmacology and Therapeutics in Nursing.* New York: McGraw-Hill.

Wordell, D. (1982). Should you crush that tablet? *Nursing 82, 12*(9), 78.

# Bibliography

Desyrel product information. (1981). Evansville, IN: Mead-Johnson Pharmaceutical Division.

Ludiomil product information. (1981). Summit, NJ: CIBA Pharmaceutical Company.

Xanax product information. (1981). Kalamazoo, MI: Upjohn.

# Generic Index

# Brand Name Index

427

428

# Systems Index